The Friedberg Metho Anesthesia: The Breakthrough Approach for Greater Patient Safety and Comfort

During surgery, how can your anesthesiologist know whether you're getting too much or too little anesthesia?

Traditionally, anesthesia dosages have been determined by a formula using patient body weight and past health history. In addition, anesthesiologists have been trained to assess patient comfort and sleep levels during surgery by checking vital signs like heart rate, blood pressure and blood oxygen levels.

Unfortunately, neither of these prevalent dosage and monitoring practices provides a high degree of reliability for 21st century care.

The Friedberg Method is a proven and time-tested method of determining more precisely how a patient is doing under anesthesia. As a result, it can put an end to over- or under-anesthesia—causes of severe patient discomfort, disorientation, dementia, or even death.

Goldilocks Anesthesia adds a brain monitor to the Friedberg Method. The brain monitor allows the anesthesiologist to know with certainty whether more or less anesthesia is needed. The brain monitor also provides a numerically reproducible number below which the patient can have surgical stimulation without pain.

In addition to outstanding patient comfort, The Friedberg Method of Goldilocks Anesthesia's record of safety has been nothing short of phenomenal:

- NO pulmonary embolisms (deadly blood clots to the lungs),
- NO patient deaths (like Donde West or Stephanie Kuleba),
- NO cardiac arrests (or near death experiences like Tameka Foster),
- NO negative pressure pulmonary edema or aspiration,
- NO 911 calls, and
- NO hospital admissions for postoperative nausea and vomiting (PONV) or pain management

It is so safe that the US military uses it on wounded soldiers in the forward MASH units, a development that earned Dr. Friedberg a US Congressional award.

Getting Over Going Under explains The Friedberg Method of Goldilocks Anesthesia in detail. It outlines how you can have your anesthesiologist more effectively keep you or your loved ones sedated and comfortable using 21st century care and it also reveals the shortcomings of 20th century anesthesia. It details the reasons for patient discomfort and worrisome side effects and how they can be eliminated. And it clearly shows what *you*, the patient can do to promote having your anesthesiologist use Goldilocks Anesthesia for cosmetic and other surgeries.

The Friedberg Method was developed in 1992 and enhanced with the addition of the brain monitor to become Goldilocks anesthesia. More than 5,000 of Dr. Friedberg's patients—and he, himself, when he had hip surgery—have enjoyed its many benefits. If you or a loved one are facing surgery of any kind, this book will assist you in assuring the safest and best possible outcome with your anesthesia experience.

Read this book and take the knowledge on its pages to your doctor so that you can greatly benefit from having a brain monitor used when anesthesia is needed.

* Dr. Friedberg has absolutely no financial connection with brain monitor manufacturers or anesthetic drug producers.

About the Author

Barry Friedberg, MD, has been a board certified anesthesiologist for over three decades.

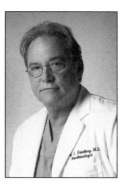

The Friedberg Method was developed in 1992 and enhanced with the addition of the brain monitor in 1997 to become Goldilocks Anesthesia. Goldilocks Anesthesia allows anesthesiologists to confidently dispense "not too much, not too little, but just the right dosage" of anesthesia. For applying his method to wounded soldiers on the combat field, Dr. Friedberg received a US Congressional award.

Dr. Friedberg is a prolific writer, passionate speaker and founder of the non-profit Goldilocks Foundation. He lives with his wife, Shelley, and his 120-pound Golden Retriever, Montgomery, in Southern California. He practices throughout the region, and speaks across the country and around the globe on the benefits of putting The Friedberg Method of Goldilocks Anesthesia into practice with measurable and repeatable results.

GETTING OVER
GOING UNDER

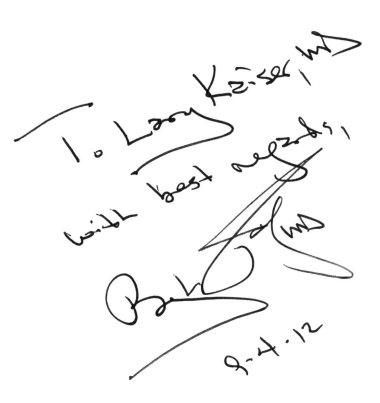

To Larry Kaiser MD
with best regards,

Barry [signature] MD

8-4-12

GETTING OVER
GOING UNDER

5 Things
You **MUST** Know
before
Anesthesia

BARRY L. FRIEDBERG M.D.

GP

Goldilocks Press
Newport Beach, CA

Goldilocks Press
P.O. Box 10336
Newport Beach, CA 92658
Phone: 949-233-8845
Fax: 949-760-9444

Printed in the United States of America

Publisher's Cataloguing-in-Publication

Friedberg, Barry L., 1948-

Getting over going under : 5 things you must know before anesthesia / Barry Friedberg. -- 1st ed. -- Newport Beach, Calif. : Goldilocks Press, c2010.

p. ; cm.

ISBN: 978-0-9829169-0-2

1. Anesthesia. 2. Anesthesia--Complications--Prevention. 3. Anesthesiology. I. Title.

RD82 .F75 2010   2010911561
617.9/6--dc22   1009

Cover Photograph and Author Photograph: Jurgen Reisch

All proceeds from the sale of this book go to support the public education mission of the non-profit Goldilocks Foundation.

*To my wife, Shelley. This book could
not have been completed without her
love and unselfish support. My life would not be
as wonderful and my work not nearly
as meaningful without her in it.*

Table of Contents

Part 3: A Patient's Bill of Rights

Wake Up,
Don't Throw Up!

Whenever going into the hospital for surgery, be it major or relatively minor, most of us worry about going under the knife. But it's not the knife we should be so worried about; our concern should be *going under* in the first place.

In fact, a recent American Society of Anesthesiologists' survey revealed that 75% of people had anesthesia fears and 25% would consider postponing their surgery because of those fears.

As a patient, we may speak with our doctors several times before a surgery; we know our surgeon and are comfortable with him. We trust his credentials, his expertise, and his experience—or we wouldn't be under his care in the first place. But when's the last time you spoke with, let alone met, your anesthesiologist?

Maybe he comes in a few minutes before he's about to put you under—maybe not. Even if he does, do you understand half of what he's telling you as he runs through his protocol? Do you know when he's going to start? Or how you'll feel when he's through with you? The truly shocking part of this equation is that your anesthesiologist typically knows as little about you as you do about him!

That's because there is no scientific formula to determine just how much anesthesia to give you. Yes, your anesthesiologist can get close to determining just how many drugs to give you to keep you sedated during your surgery—typically by factoring in your weight, your age, and whether or not you smoke or drink and how often. But ultimately the resulting equation is merely an elaborate piece of guesswork, no more scientific than the comical huckster who guesses your weight at the carnival!

What typically happens as a result of this unscientific method is that your anesthesiologist either prescribes too much medication … or not enough. Now, we've all heard the horror stories of patients who aren't given enough anesthesia, waking up before their surgery is complete and suffering severe pain. Since this is obviously traumatic, most anesthesiologists err on the side of caution. How? By giving you too much anesthesia instead of too little. Unfortunately, the side effects of too many drugs can be as catastrophic—though not as readily visible—as not administering enough.

Too much anesthesia can make us groggy when we wake up from surgery, increase nausea, and instigate headaches, but these are easily remedied and overcome in a hospital setting.

Unfortunately, along with these less severe side effects, over-medication can trigger an Alzheimer's-like dementia and that *doesn't* go away. Suddenly you have tremendous social costs. It's tragic because when you damage the brain to the degree of creating dementia, there is no undoing it.

These symptoms may sound uncommon, perhaps because you've never experienced them before, but in fact every year in this country 99.9 percent of up to 40 million people are routinely exposed to overmedication. [*Source*: 2004 Emory University study.] Patients over the age of fifty are especially susceptible to the risks of dementia and death from routine anesthesia overmedication. In fact, 2,255 patients died between 1999 and 2005 from routine anesthesia overmedication—nearly one a day! [*Source*: Li, April 2009 *Anesthesiology*]

And therein lies the dilemma American anesthesiologists have been dealing with for decades before the advent of practical direct brain monitoring: Either we give too little anesthesia and run the risk of a patient "coming to" during significant surgery, or we give too much anesthesia and run the risk of damaging our patients' brains. It's no easy choice.

The worst part of this nightmare scenario is that it doesn't have to be this way. Typically during surgery your anesthesiologist will routinely monitor your vital signs: heartbeat, breathing, blood pressure, and so on. But unless you ask for it by name, anesthesiologists do not routinely *monitor your brain*.

Why not? Heart rate, blood pressure, and breathing changes tell the anesthesiologist a great deal about you from the neck down, but anesthesia medicates you from the neck up! So why measure what the brain controls (i.e., the neck down) when you can literally measure the brain itself? If we want to avoid brain damage, it makes more sense for anesthesiologists to monitor the brain! Your right as an informed consumer/patient is to be sure this is going to be done—or to go elsewhere where it is practiced.

You might think it's expensive, too technical, or even impossible to measure the brain during surgery, but that's not so. In fact, for as little as $20, hospitals can safely, effectively, and accurately measure your brain before and during surgery to make sure that you get exactly the right amount of anesthesia for any procedure—every time.

So why aren't more hospitals doing it? It all boils down to politics. (And really, doesn't everything?) For one, the technology is so readily available, the application of the device so easy, and the device itself so inexpensive that no one is making any money doing it.

Using a brain monitor, your anesthesiologist will often lessen the drug dosage by up to *30 percent per procedure*! The major pharmaceutical companies (aka Big Pharma) are absolutely "unhappy" about a device that could cut into their sales so drastically. Imagine losing 30 percent of your drug sales every time a patient undergoes surgery. Naturally, they push hard to sell more, not fewer, patent-protected drugs and subtly reward doctors for *not* using this simple, affordable device.

And let's not underestimate a doctor's medical training. To *unlearn* all he or she has been taught in nearly a dozen years of college, medical school, residency, and additional training is a tall order, and one few doctors willingly embrace. So that status quo remains the status quo, and as a result, you—the surgical patient—will on average receive a dosage of anesthetic drugs that is 30 percent higher than you really need because you never knew to ask to have your brain monitored during surgery.

Approximately 60 percent of American hospitals have brain monitors, but the monitors are only implemented 20 percent of the time. Another reason your hospital may not encourage brain monitoring is that they are only in the "business" of acute care. As long as you go home alive, they have met *their* benchmark. The chronic condition of your brain after overmedication with anesthesia remains *your* problem (and society's cost) for the rest of your life.

My name is Dr. Barry Friedberg, and my career is the medical practice of anesthesia. My formal anesthesia training was at Stanford (1975-1977) after which I passed my boards to become a Diplomate of the American Board of Anesthesiology or a board certified anesthesiologist (1980). Today, I run the not-for-profit Goldilocks Foundation.

Inside *Getting Over Going Under* you will discover the many dangers of over- and under-medicating, the simple tools you need for arming yourself with information, a complete Patients' Bill of Rights plus the nine essential questions you must ask your surgeon before surgery.

My goal is to make sure you awaken from anesthesia as the same person who went to under; i.e. keeping all the mental 'marbles' with which you started!

Barry L. Friedberg, M.D.
Corona del Mar, California

PART 1

*The Goldilocks Principle—
Measuring Is Better Than Guessing*

Chapter 1

Why Old Anesthesia Techniques Don't Work

Over the past 13 years of advocating brain monitored anesthesia, I've heard from many relatives and friends about loved ones who have awakened from anesthesia not quite the same person they were before they went under. Why? The routine overuse of anesthetic drugs.

When you watch a TV show like *House* or walk through a hospital, you see an over-abundance of equipment and monitors, so most people figure that something as logical as a brain monitor would be in use when doctors administer general anesthesia. But they aren't widely implemented at all, and many patients don't realize they can ask their anesthesiologist to use one.

And they should if they want to wake up from their anesthetic with the same number of mental "marbles" with which they went "under." This chapter describes why the traditional practice of over-anesthetizing patients is no longer valid, let alone safe, for modern, twenty-first century consumers such as yourself.

In your continuing role as a more informed medical consumer, it is vital that you know the truth about anesthesia as it is practiced today and the bright promise it holds for the future—IF you and I can band together and demand brain monitors in every hospital, for every surgery, for every patient, every time.

More Is Not Always More: *The Case for Less*

According to the U.S. Department of Health and Human Services, an estimated 53.3 million surgical and nonsurgical procedures are performed during 34.7 million ambulatory surgery visits each year. That's a lot of surgery, and a lot of people being put under general anesthesia *without knowing all the risks*.

Without a brain monitor, anesthesiology is not an exact science. This is shocking to many patients, but it's true. Anesthesiologists ask whether you smoke or drink, how often, what you weigh, and how tall you are so that they can "guesstimate" the amount of anesthesia to give you.

This inexact science is the great failure of anesthesia; not because it exists, but because it doesn't *have* to exist. Simple, modern, effective, and inexpensive technology exists to more scientifically and accurately measure the exact amount of anesthesia you need, but even the most modern hospitals and most qualified anesthesiologists still don't take advantage of it; this chapter will tell you why.

Please understand before we proceed that it is NOT my goal to make anesthesiologists look bad. These are my colleagues, co-workers, and comrades, after all. I have made my career in anesthesiology and everything I do is to improve the state of anesthesiology in this country and, as often as possible, around the world. However, as a doctor my first loyalty is to my patient, and if I've found something that helps ease my patient's transition from surgery to recovery, then I'm duty-bound to support them, even at the expense of my comrades' feelings.

One such way many anesthesiologists practice their profession at the expense of, rather than in support of, their patients is failing to measure how much anesthesia to prescribe. Unfortunately, because of this inexact science, most doctors figure it is better to give the patient more than they need in order to make sure they don't wake up during the operation. After explaining the virtues of fewer drugs to some colleagues, one of them remarked, "That's nice, but the more drugs I give, the better I feel."

This attitude likely reflects this anesthesiologist treating his own anxieties instead of measuring what his patients actually need! Of course, no one in the healthcare food chain is opposed to using more drugs, as that is a large part of the revenue stream for all involved parties, i.e., hospitals and Big Pharma (America's powerful drug makers). In a very real sense, the patient's interest comes last, preceded by the pharmaceutical company's interest and the hospital's interest. Everyone aside from you, the patient, is interested in the same thing: profit.

There's an old saying, *"If it ain't broke, don't fix it."* Well, in anesthesiology, many doctors have always given more drugs than less, having never been encouraged to do anything else, and figure, *"Why rock the boat if nobody's dying?"* And that's just the point of this book; before you met me, you likely didn't realize there was an alternative to too much, let alone too little, anesthesia.

Now you know that you can help inform anesthesiologists all over the world that there is a better way, and it stems from one of the oldest known fairytales! (But more on that later.)

By using a brain monitor to guide anesthesia dosing, each patient becomes an "open book test" instead of "a mystery to be solved."

Doctors would be able to use a more exact (and smaller) dosage and be safer as a result. Instead of using too little or too much, they'd use a dosage that is just right, hence my reference to Goldilocks anesthesia with my foundation's name.

The risks of being over-anesthetized are many, including delirium, long-term dementia, memory loss, and even death. Doctors, hospitals, and pharmaceutical companies may be aware of the dangers and statistics of over-usage, but most patients are not. Unfortunately, not enough research has been conducted on anesthesia overdosing because without widespread use of brain monitors during surgery, there is no way to pinpoint whether anesthesia is statistically a culprit even though common sense would indicate a high probability.

Preoperatively, a mentally normal patient who becomes less than the thinking person he or she was after being anesthetized makes a good case for a *res ipsa loquitor* (Latin for "the thing speaks for itself"). Anesthetics medicate the brain. Why not at least suspect that too much anesthesia might be the cause of a sudden onset of dementia after anesthesia when there was none beforehand? Is this proposition not self-evident?

The risk of overmedication is the reason why I urge all my patients to ask if their anesthesiologist uses a brain monitor during the surgery and to ask for a different anesthesiologist if the one assigned to them doesn't use one or, for that matter, doesn't know what one is!

What's that? You didn't realize you could ask for another anesthesiologist? The fact is you have many choices before undergoing surgery, and we will explore all of them in later chapters of this book. For now, though, it is important to approach your surgery and anesthesia armed with the facts you'll need to be sure you wake up the same person you were before anesthesia!

The message at hand seems simple and prudent enough monitor the brain during surgery, not just the signals put out by the brain. But this message has not been adopted by my profession or the healthcare industry *because the major players don't make money from its use.* Hospitals don't even have billing codes for the $20 disposable sensor for a brain monitor, and the pharmaceutical companies sponsoring all the junkets for doctors aren't fond of them because they invariably result in the use of smaller amounts of the drugs they sell.

Again, please understand that I don't make any money from trying to spread this message. I don't have a "secret deal" with the monitor manufacturers, and I don't have an axe to grind with the drug companies. In fact, the promotion of my crusade has cost me professional relationships as well as money out of my own pocket.

I am just tired of the primary task of my profession being not to kill patients. Instead, we should focus on caring for the patients and understanding the long-term risks of overmedicating patients in surgery. We should implement every modern tool available to keep them healthy and reduce unnecessary risks through the entire treatment process.

Voice Your Concerns About Over-Anesthesia!

If you think waking up with pain is the top concern of patients undergoing surgery, think again. According to a recent study on anesthesia, patients listed vomiting, NOT pain, as the number one postoperative condition they would like to avoid. The medical community knows over-anesthetizing is a frequent cause of such nausea, so it's time for my colleagues to adopt new technology that may allow anesthesiologists to more accurately administer dosages.

Despite the dangers of either under- or over-anesthetizing a patient, the device, which measures brain activity to determine the state of a patient's consciousness, is only employed in 20 percent of hospital operating rooms despite the fact that 60 percent of hospitals have the equipment. This is concerning because this equipment can greatly improve a patient's overall post-surgical experience. We obviously don't want to under-medicate, but patients have indicated that they consider a fast and comfortable recovery to also be very important.

One device for brain monitoring, the bispectral (BIS) index, measures brain activity and consciousness during sedation and general anesthesia. In the past, anesthesiologists have monitored heart rate and blood pressure changes. Keeping an eye on the heart is essential for assessing how the *body* is reacting to the anesthesia. But the BIS allows us to monitor the organ we are trying to sedate—*the brain*. Hand in hand, the two methods allow us to better gauge the patient's state of sleep and overall health. FDA approved in 1996, BIS has also been proven to work in more than 3,500 published scientific studies. It makes sense to add it routinely to the operating room monitors.

My concern is that many hospitals and clinics might be putting the bottom line before patient care. The relentless focus on the cost of healthcare is causing administrators to make some decisions at the expense of patients. However, allowing anesthesiologists to do their jobs in the best possible way will ultimately reduce costs. If we can make the anesthesia dosage more accurate, the patient will recover quicker, helping to eliminate unnecessarily lengthy, overnight stays or even re-admission for control of postoperative nausea and vomiting (PONV) or post-op pain.

Anesthesia is still not an exact science. Traditionally, anesthesiologists would medicate a patient much like a person makes a pot of coffee. You measure six cups of water, then six spoonfuls of coffee grounds and then you throw in an extra spoonful for the pot. BIS eliminates the extra spoonful by providing information that allows for a more exact measure of medicine. An appropriate dosage typically leads to a more rapid recovery, and that's the whole point.

Forty million patients undergo surgery with general anesthesia or deep sedation each year in the United States. Experts expect this number to rise due to an increase in cosmetic surgeries following the tragedies of September 11. Because people saw how uncertain life could be, they stopped putting off doing things for themselves, including elective beauty procedures. And that has led to an increase in the number of people going under.

Neither Awake or in a Coma: *The Power of Film*

The movie *Awake* is a psychological thriller that tells the story of a man who suffers "anesthetic awareness" and finds himself awake and aware, but paralyzed, during heart surgery.

Can you imagine? The fear of waking up during surgery has made for a compelling movie and great box office and continues to be a fear of my patients long after the movie's release several years ago. But it's not my first run-in with movie-induced anesthesia panic!

It has been thirty years since Robin Cook's book *Coma* captured and terrified the American public's imagination. *Coma* is the gripping story of patients who check into a hospital for "minor" surgery and never wake up again. Long after the book and movie, I still had patients extremely reluctant to have surgery in Room 8, the site of *Coma's* (fictional) dastardly deeds!

In pointing out the difference between fact and fiction, back in 1977, the anesthesia profession was seven short years away from the kind of technology that would have obviated the premise of *Coma* (i.e., inflicting the lack of oxygen to produce the vegetative state in patients so they could be harvested for organ transplants). That technology, the pulse oximeter, was introduced in 1984. Pulse oximetry was deemed "a standard of care" by the American Society of Anesthesiologists (ASA) a full six years later. Primarily serving as a political organization, the ASA sometimes lags behind reasonable clinical practice. After all, why wouldn't you want to know instantaneously if your patient had adequate oxygen in their blood?

History repeated itself in 2007, when the movie *Awake* needlessly terrified the American public, again. This time the technology that nullifies the premise of the movie has been available since 1996, when the FDA approved its use. Again, why wouldn't you want to know *how* asleep your patient is?

No technology is perfect, even level of consciousness monitors. The prototype is the bispectral (BIS) index monitor. A published scientific study (2004) showed it was 82 percent *less* likely for patients to remain awake when their anesthesiologist believed they were asleep. Why, then, have considerable numbers of anesthesia providers been reluctant to adopt BIS monitoring? Because measuring the brain's response to anesthetics challenges the deeply held belief system that heart rate and blood pressure changes are reliable guides to the depth of anesthesia.

These changes are now known to be notoriously unreliable guides to your brain's response to anesthetics. Heart rate and blood pressure changes are merely bodily readings signaled by the brain, but why get diluted (or "downstream") information when you can get direct signals from the brain itself merely by monitoring the brain during surgery?

In the well-known fairytale, Goldilocks finally finds porridge that is not too hot (Poppa Bear), not too cold (Momma Bear), but just right (Baby Bear). Goldilocks anesthesia is where patients are neither over-anesthetized nor under-anesthetized, but just rightly anesthetized.

The consequences of overdosing may be even more sinister than under-dosing. It is not uncommon for relatives of elderly patients to observe that they are "mentally not quite the same" after their anesthesia. The fancy doctor term for losing some of one's 'marbles' is postoperative cognitive dysfunction (POCD). Many believe, as do I, that POCD may also be a function of anesthetic overmedication. Given its history with pulse oximetry, the public should not rely on the ASA to insist that BIS monitoring be a standard of care in the 21st century.

The greatest good that may come from *Awake* is the groundswell of public opinion demanding routine brain monitoring for general anesthesia.

Consider the (Direct) Source

Most patients tolerate their anesthetic experience despite the care they receive rather than because of it.

The public has been taught that "doctors know best," and as a result, they put their lives in doctors' hands (often) without question. Likewise, most doctors rely on what they've been taught to guide their hands as well.

Case in point: anesthesiologists (and nurse anesthetists) have traditionally been taught to medicate patients on a per-kilogram of body weight to begin the patient's anesthesia. After the patient is asleep, subsequent medication doses are then adjusted primarily based upon changes in heart rate and blood pressure. However, the object of the anesthetic agents is to medicate the patient's brain, not their heart rate and blood pressure. Before 1996, to ensure patients were actually asleep, the anesthesia provider was obliged to overmedicate for fear of under-medicating.

The first level of consciousness or brain monitor was FDA approved in 1996. Although several competitors exist in the marketplace, none has presented any studies demonstrating superiority to the original device. Conversely, over 3,500 scientific papers attest to its utility.

A force for change must be created by greater public awareness of the dangers of excessive anesthesia. For maximum patient safety, brain monitoring *absolutely* must be the standard of care in the twenty-first century.

Chapter 2

Knowledge Conquers
Anesthesia Fears

Fear is your greatest enemy before your surgery. In fact, a recent American Society of Anesthesiologists' survey revealed that 75% of people had anesthesia fears and 25% would consider postponing their surgery because of those fears.

Whether conscious or subconscious, the fears you carry with you on your day of surgery (aka your emotional baggage) are not something our anesthetic drugs can control. You must learn to be the master of your own emotions. The knowledge you will gain from this chapter should help you conquer your fears.

As the recent ASA survey documented, anesthesia fears abound. Even I, a 33-year veteran of administering anesthesia to others, was not at all excited about the prospect of having anesthesia *given to me!*

When I needed to have my own hip replaced in May 2008, you can be very sure I absolutely insisted on the use of a brain monitor to ensure I woke up the same person that I was before surgery. Near as I can tell, I did or I wouldn't be writing this book for you!

Where do anesthesia fears come from?

1. Personal bad experience with difficulty waking up or throwing up after waking up

2. Personal bad experience with pain after surgery that needed strong narcotic painkillers like morphine or Vicodin®

3. Friends or family members who have experienced issues #1 and/or 2

4. The movie *Awake,* or other media accounts of patients being awake when their anesthesiologist thought they were asleep (anesthesia awareness fears)

5. Family or friends' death during (or after) anesthesia

6. Friends or family who were not sure who they were when they woke up from anesthesia (anesthesia overmedication)

7. Friends or family who were never quite the same person they were before their surgery and anesthesia (anesthesia overmedication)

I started the Goldilocks Foundation to alert the public about the *critical* need for brain monitors when going under anesthesia for surgery. However, the Friedberg Method of Goldilocks Anesthesia entails far more than directly measuring your brain's response to anesthetics. By explaining my Friedberg Method of Goldilocks Anesthesia, all of your fears about experiencing anesthesia in the 21st century should be banished.

Before 1984 and the introduction of the pulse oximeter, death related to anesthesia happened in about one of every 10,000 surgeries. After oximetry became commonplace, death rates plummeted to about one in every 250,000 surgeries. According to a 2009 JAMA article, during 1999-2005, *the overall annual motor vehicle death rate did not change substantially* (about 15.4 per 100,000 population). Putting death from anesthesia in a larger perspective, it appears that driving to your hospital has a higher risk than having anesthesia for your surgery.

In the late 1980s, the most wonderful anesthesia drug in the last hundred years was brought to the North American market. That drug was the milky white-colored propofol (Diprivan®). It replaced our old friend, thiopental or Pentothal,® the so-called "truth serum." In reality, no one ever stayed awake long enough to tell any truths under Pentothal.®

Why is propofol the most wonderful anesthetic drug? First, its quick onset and quick recovery profile made it an ideal drug for sedation and anesthesia. Estimates are that nearly 80 percent of surgery is performed on an outpatient basis. As the trend toward outpatient surgery accelerated in the 1990s, propofol became immensely popular despite its cost. However, now that propofol is generic, cost is no longer an issue. The immense popularity of propofol makes the current (2010) shortage guaranteed to be short-lived.

Propofol has also been found to be a powerful anti-nausea drug. In 1999, a statistically validated survey of what you, the patient, most desired to avoid was published. To no one's surprise in the non-academic world, throwing up after waking up (emesis) was the least desired outcome (with #3 being nauseated without throwing up). Together #1 and #3 make up what is frequently referred to as postoperative nausea and vomiting (PONV).

Sadly, the companion survey done with anesthesiologists showed *they* thought a patient most wanted to avoid pain. Pain was actually ranked #4 in your survey. Most of you anticipate some discomfort after surgery. Probably what you were trying to tell the anesthesiologists was you did not want to have "salt rubbed in your wounds" by throwing up in addition to your anticipated discomfort.

Propofol is an anti-oxidant while the "stinky gases" (isoflurane, sevoflurane, and desflurane) are oxidizing agents. Stinky gases are known to raise your blood markers for inflammation (C-reactive proteins) and may even contribute to the growth of cancers beyond their original site (metastasis).

Additionally, during surgery, stinky gases do not prevent your brain from *receiving* the painful messages. Accumulation of the pain signals in your brain *during* surgery is called the "wind-up" phenomenon. The brain winds up in response to the non-stop barrage of incoming pain signals while you are unconscious and helpless. More on this in Chapters Eight and Nine.

When you wake up in recovery, the wind-up phenomenon often leaves you in need of strong narcotic pain killers like morphine or Vicodin.® (Translation: postoperative pain comes from *intra*-operative pain—a radical concept.) Strong narcotic painkillers are also recognized as a leading cause of PONV.

Most anesthesiologists (and nurse anesthetists) continue to routinely administer either or both stinky gases and strong narcotic painkillers (emetogenic agents). In *Miller's Anesthesia*, the top anesthesia textbook for the last twenty-five years, the world's leading authority on PONV has clearly stated that as long as emetogenic agents are given, the use of anti-nausea drugs is of *limited* usefulness, while citing my 1999 paper that showed the *lowest* PONV rate (0.6%) in the anesthesia literature without the use of anti-nausea drugs (with a sample size of 1,264 patients).

Goldilocks anesthesia relies on the brain monitor to show your anesthesiologist a reproducible number (i.e., less than 75) at which a "nifty" 50 mg dose of ketamine can be given, keeping you from feeling any pain while you are anesthetized, yet without giving you bad dreams. (Ketamine is a very interesting drug with a checkered past. There is more about this fascinating drug in the next chapter.)

The difference between using ketamine *before* surgery stimulation is most readily understood by a common experience at the dentist's office. When your teeth are numbed before dental work, you typically feel some discomfort or pain *before* your teeth go numb. Surprisingly, that is exactly what happens under anesthesia *without* pre-treatment with ketamine even though you are asleep and unable to respond.

With the ketamine pre-treatment, your brain never gets the information because that initial pain signal never arrives. *Your brain cannot "wind-up" from information it never receives!* Sometimes I use the expression that ketamine puts your brain on "call waiting" while your body is having surgery. The fancy doctor term for this phenomenon is preemptive analgesia or not hurting you in the first place.

Not only have more than 5,000 of my patients over the past eighteen years received this fantastic benefit, but I also did when I had my hip replaced. The only difference between my spinal anesthetic with brain-monitored propofol sedation and the treatment of hundreds of other patients at this hospital was that I received a dose of 50 mg ketamine three minutes before stimulation. While I cannot guarantee the same experience for you, I had no pain for four days after my hip replacement!

Last but not least, propofol is a "happy" drug. Patients enjoy the experience of being put to "sleep" with it and the feeling of waking up from it.

But, given quickly, in a typical "go-to-sleep" dose (50-100 milligrams), propofol often causes you to stop breathing and your tongue to fall back in your throat, blocking the air from getting in and out of your lungs. Your anesthesiologist is well trained to support your breathing, but why interfere with your ability in the first place?

To avoid this potential hazard, between 1992 and 1994, I began using propofol to *gradually* induce anesthesia to maintain a patient's ability to breathe on their own. When patients awakened, I always asked them how they felt about their anesthesia. Every single patient over that two-year period always said the same thing: "The best part was the 'going to sleep' part."

I had no frame of reference to understand what my patients were telling me. After two years of hearing the same thing, the lightbulb went off in my head. Propofol is a happy drug. Patients liked it. Long before Michael Jackson cried for his "milk," I already knew more than 5,000 of my patients enjoyed their anesthetic. In summary, my Friedberg Method of Goldilocks Anesthesia is to:

1. *Measure the brain*

2. *Preempt the pain*

3. *Emetic ('gag me') drugs abstain*

Chapter 3

Facing the Establishment— Getting the Goldilocks Method

Now that you know what the Friedberg Method of Goldilocks Anesthesia can do for you, how do you get it?

Obviously, the first person you will encounter will be your surgeon. And the first item on your list of questions will typically *not* be, "What kind of anesthesia do you give your patients?" The really big question on your mind will be *"Doctor, do I really have to have this surgery?"*

Unless you are a family member or friend of mine who has listened to me talk about Goldilocks anesthesia, you will be completely focused on the body part on which you are going to have surgery. You are rightly concerned about the results of your surgery. If you are going under for this surgery, you are putting your most precious, irreplaceable asset at risk—your brain!

The function of the Goldilocks Foundation is to raise your awareness of the value of waking up from surgery the same person you were before surgery. If you've read this far, you probably understand that *there are major and minor surgeries, but every anesthetic is major!*

Surgeons who operate in their office or a surgery center usually control who gives anesthesia to their patients and what kind of anesthesia is going to be provided. These surgeons are most likely to be able to accommodate your desire for Goldilocks anesthesia. Unfortunately, most surgeons operate either in a hospital or a surgery center. Many times these facilities have their anesthesia staff under contract. Thus, the anesthesiologists may be indifferent to the request of the surgeon for Goldilocks anesthesia.

The task of contacting the anesthesia staff will then become your responsibility. Often this is not easily accomplished. Your anesthesiologist is frequently occupied during daytime hours giving anesthesia to other patients. Sometimes this task can more efficiently be accomplished via email.

Because of its numerous advantages (see Chapter 2), propofol-based anesthesia has become very popular. So a good starting point would be to find out if this type of anesthesia is administered at the place you plan to have your surgery and, of course, who will be giving it—an anesthesiologist, a nurse anesthetist or an anesthesiologist supervised anesthesia assistant. These questions should not put anyone on the defensive. But if they do, you should consider *having your surgery elsewhere!*

Should you do decide to go elsewhere, consider downloading the administrator letter from www.drbarryfriedberg.com to send to the facility you did not go to letting that person know why.

This action on your part will help create the force for change that will bring about universal brain monitoring for anyone going under.

The next big question is about brain monitoring. You may hear, "We don't think that's necessary." However, the point is not for you to engage in a discussion about beliefs. You are not interested in the beliefs of the anesthesia staff. You are vitally interested in the best result for your brain after anesthesia, period.

Instead of trying to convince an anesthesia professional of the worthiness of brain monitoring, try kicking this person in the wallet! Politely explain that unless you can be assured a brain monitor will be used, you will have your surgeon take your surgery somewhere where a brain monitor will be. This kind of dialogue is the only way you can avoid the unnecessary and common risks of anesthesia overmedication as well as the extremely rare risk of under-medication.

If you have gotten this far in your conversation with your anesthesiologist, you have secured two-thirds of the Friedberg Method of Goldilocks Anesthesia. Getting your "nifty fifty"—or 50 milligrams of ketamine after you are anesthetized and three minutes BEFORE your surgeon stimulates you—will be the biggest challenge you will face. Unless this hospital or surgery center has adopted the Friedberg Method of Goldilocks Anesthesia, you will undoubtedly hear what a "bad" drug ketamine is and why they don't think it's a good idea to give it to adults.

The way to defeat this argument is as follows: "If your patients still need narcotic painkillers after surgery, but Goldilocks patients only take Tylenol, don't you think this 'nifty fifty' is worth considering, especially since I am asking you politely?" If a concern is still expressed to you, try saying that as long as your brain monitor is showing a propofol level below 75, you won't have any bad dreams but have a 5 percent chance of having pleasant colorful dreams.

I never promised you this task would be easy or readily accepted by your surgeon or anesthesiologist. However, if you believe that it is far better to have surgery by measuring your brain, not hurting you while you are anesthetized and not getting drugs that can make you sick to your stomach, then all of this effort will be more than worthwhile.

If you still face resistance to this very reasonable idea, feel free to refer your surgeon and anesthesiologist to www.drfriedberg.com (Ch. 1 of Anesthesia in Cosmetic Surgery, Tables 1-6 through 1-9 free) and www.goldilocksanesthesia.com for more information about Goldilocks anesthesia or contact me personally via email at drfriedberg@drfriedberg.com.

Your friends and family will be pleasantly surprised when they see you after surgery with Goldilocks anesthesia. Expect comments such as "You don't even look like you've had surgery!" Believe me, when you can have surgery, wake up feeling great, not sick to your stomach or in pain, the same person who went under, you will be *Getting Over Going Under*"!

Chapter 4

Why My Crusade & Goldilocks Foundation

I am an anesthesiologist because I do not want you, my patient, to suffer. I am also an anesthesiologist because *I* have suffered from anesthesia, not once but twice, in my youth. Your pain is also my pain. Your suffering is my suffering. I empathize with every one of my patients' trials to thrive after their surgeries. Before anesthesia, surgery was the great societal leveler, kings and commoners alike suffered. With Goldilocks anesthesia, no one should have to suffer.

Despite my best efforts, the first twenty years of my anesthesia practice resulted in patients needing powerful narcotic painkillers after surgery. Most of the time, I administered stinky gases and narcotics, the so-called emetogenic agents that account for most PONV. Only when I was presented with the challenge to provide anesthesia *without emetogenic drugs* did the propofol ketamine sedation or the Friedberg Method evolve. (Emeotgenic drugs are the intravenous narcotics and stinky gases.) Only after I faced *my* need to have anesthesia did I come to understand that you (the public) deserve to know the problem, be offered the solution, and receive your call to action.

Over the past eighteen years, I gave the "nifty fifty" to more than five thousand of you and was extremely gratified with the results. (The "nifty fifty" is 50 milligrams of ketamine three minutes before stimulation. Preferably, the stimulation should be the local anesthetic injection of the skin your surgeon is about to be cut. Fifty is the magic dose of ketamine for adults. Nifty describes the obviously better results!)

Firsthand, I saw the entire spectrum of cosmetic surgery cases performed without PONV, pain or delirium, dementia or death. My colleagues in anesthesia have always been quick to dismiss the Friedberg Method of Goldilocks Anesthesia because I only administered it for *those* types of surgery.

Two years ago, in 2008, after I experienced the same benefit from the "nifty fifty" with *my* hip replacement surgery, I understood my colleagues were totally wrong about the Friedberg Method of Goldilocks Anesthesia.

None of the nurses who cared for me in the hospital ward when I returned from surgery could believe I had my hip replaced. None of them knew I had received the "nifty fifty," yet every one of them independently remarked to me, "You don't look like you've had surgery. We've *never* seen a hip look like you!" Clearly, my Friedberg Method of Goldilocks Anesthesia will work for any surgery, not only the cosmetic ones!

I am frequently asked why something as self-evident as measuring the effects of anesthesia directly from your brain is still not a commonplace practice or a standard of twenty-first century anesthesia care. While this question is simple and straightforward, the answer is complex, many layered, and not readily susceptible to sound bites.

We know from the Biblical accounts of the prophets' struggle to affect change in human behavior that change is the hardest thing one human can ever hope to promote. All people resist change. It disturbs the status quo, is perceived as a threat, and forces one to think or act differently. Change is always resisted until a force for that change becomes too much to fight.

Only an informed public demand can create the force for change for brain monitoring as a 21st century standard of anesthesia care!

Physicians are notoriously resistant to changing their practices. Doctors, like your anesthesiologist who deals with life and death daily, all tend to believe that what stands between you and the pearly gates is the way we give your anesthesia. Most anesthesiologists feel that as long as you don't die from the anesthesia, they have done their job. That was an acceptable attitude in the twentieth century. Merely surviving anesthesia is no longer acceptable in the twenty-first century. Today, we absolutely insist on waking up the same person we were before we went under.

But what else stands in the way of widespread acceptance of brain monitoring as the standard of twenty-first century anesthesia care? Perhaps even more potent than the money issues discussed in chapter one is the difficulty in abandoning the belief system that heart rate and blood pressure changes are tied in some way to your brain's response to anesthesia drugs.

Although it's hard to believe, this belief system is *still* being taught to anesthesia trainees in some of America's most prestigious centers—although it has been known for some time that those signs are notoriously unreliable. Your anesthesiologist and hospital are only involved with your acute care while you're in their facility. Such things as how well you can balance your checkbook or relate to your friends and family are not on their radar.

Only you will be forced to live with the possible long-term consequences of your short-term care.

Chapter 5

The Michael Jackson Death— A Predictable, Avoidable Tragedy

In June 2009, Michael Jackson was transported via ambulance to Los Angeles' Cedars Sinai Hospital and pronounced dead. Although legal proceedings for involuntary manslaughter are still pending against Jackson's physician, Conrad Murray, enough facts have been publicly disclosed to make me feel that this chapter was a needed addition.

Propofol is the last of a series of drugs Dr. Murray admitted to giving Jackson. Murray publically admitted being "out of the room" shortly after giving Jackson the propofol. Propofol is the drug the LA coroner declared was the cause of Jackson's death. Murray claims to be a cardiologist. He may have been qualified to intravenously administer members of the class of drugs known as benzodiazepines or "benzos," but was most assuredly out of his depth of knowledge, training, and experience when giving propofol.

Before I go any farther, let me emphatically state that since its 1989 introduction to the North American market, tens (if not hundreds) of millions of patients have safely received propofol (also known by its trade name as Diprivan®). Why? Because someone was watching and monitoring them, two features apparently absent in Michael Jackson's bedroom.

Also administering propofol in a person's home is not altogether different from giving anesthesia in a surgeon's office operating room. Both are remote locations and can be made safe with observation and appropriate monitoring. Although I have never given propofol in a patient's home, I have safely given it to patients for office-based elective cosmetic surgery for nearly two decades.

Using propofol to help someone fight insomnia is most definitely not among the medically recognized uses of the drug. From 1992 through 1994, I put patients to sleep for cosmetic surgery in a gradual fashion to preserve their ability to breathe. What every patient told me during this two-year period was the best part of the anesthesia was the "going to sleep" part.

I had no frame of reference to understand what my patients told me. Finally, after hearing the same accounting from every patient, it occurred to me that propofol was a "happy" drug (i.e., patients enjoyed it). In 1998, one patient was so enthusiastic about his propofol experience that he suggested that he and I open a sleep clinic for patients wanting the great propofol sleep and wake up. I told him I was confident we could make a lot of money but that the California Medical Board would not view our activities as legitimate.

So I knew about the "happy" part of the propofol long before Michael Jackson's expressed love of his propofol "milk." It was likely he became familiar with propofol as a result of the multiple cosmetic surgeries he had after his hair caught fire doing the infamous Pepsi commercial.

Propofol was introduced as a replacement for thiopental or Pentothal® and is commonly used to induce or start general anesthesia. Both thiopental and propofol can cause a stoppage of breathing if given too quickly or in too large a dose. Until recently, propofol has only been administered by dedicated, trained anesthesia providers such as anesthesiologists, nurse anesthetists, or even anesthesia assistants under supervision. When given for surgery, propofol is *always* monitored with electrocardiogram (EKG), blood pressure, and pulse oximeter (SpO_2).

Introduced in 1984, the pulse oximeter was deemed a standard of care in 1990. This device emits an audible sound that decreases as a patient's breathing becomes inadequate. The advantage of the sound is it provides information to the anesthesia provider even if that provider does not have visual contact with the monitor (i.e., if not physically present).

Recently, gastroenterologists have been using propofol sedation for colonoscopies and upper endoscopies instead of fentanyl (a powerful synthetic narcotic 100 times more powerful than morphine) and the "benzo," midazolam (Versed®). All members of the benzodiazepine family end in the letters "am," diazepam (Valium®), lorazepam (Ativan®), etc. There is a big difference between the sites of action for midzolam as compared to propofol. Midazolam acts primarily on the midbrain whereas propofol primarily affects the cortex, cerebral hemispheres, or "upper" brain.

Here is the publically known timeline for the medications Murray gave to Jackson:

- *1:30 a.m.*   *10 mg diazepam (Valium®)*
- *2:00 a.m.*   *2 mg lorezepam (Ativan®)*
- *3:00 a.m.*   *2 mg midazolam (Versed®)*
- *5:00 a.m.*   *2 mg lorazepam (Ativan®)*
- *7:30 a.m.*   *2 mg midazolam (Versed®)*
- *10:30 a.m.*   *25 mg propofol (Diprivan® or "milk")*

Brain monitors like the bispectral (BIS) index measure drug effects in the cortex. The action of propofol on Jackson's brain would have been measured by a BIS monitor independently from the benzo effect. By using such a brain measurement, the overmedication with propofol could have been avoided. Jackson's failure to breathe from the combined effects of the benzos and the propofol would have also been avoided.

When midazolam was introduced to replace the longer-acting diazepam, the drug maker supplied midazolam in the same 5-milligram concentration as diazepam. After many patients had unintentional stoppage of breathing, midazolam was reformulated in a less potent concentration. For many years, midazolam has been well known for its potential to stop breathing.

Propofol is not physically addictive, but like any substance that is pleasurable, it *is* psychologically addictive. Physical addiction is defined by withdrawal or "cold turkey" symptoms if the agent is not supplied. The first Murray folly was the notion of propofol "addiction." The second fallacious notion was attempting to "wean" Jackson from a potential propofol addiction by giving him members of the benzo family. The third and lethal folly was giving Jackson two types of drugs well known to potentially stop breathing.

In none of the published photographs of Jackson's bedroom do any safety monitors appear. Murray reportedly told police he had been using a pulse oximeter. When the police searched for it, the pulse oximeter was discovered in a closet in an adjoining room. If this account proves correct, it casts serious doubts on Conrad Murray's credibility.

While midazolam comes as 1 or 2 mg per cc concentrations, propofol comes as a 10 mg per cc preparation. Giving Jackson a 1 or 2 cc dose of midazolam would have been easy for Murray. As ill informed as Murray apparently was about intravenous sedation, his representation of giving what would have been a 2.5 cc dose of propofol is simply not credible. It is more probable that Murray had no idea exactly how much drug he gave Jackson. In any case, the amount of propofol the LA coroner found in Jackson's blood is incompatible with a 25 mg dose.

Some rumors have surfaced that Murray may try to claim someone else (like Michael himself) may have given the larger dose of propofol that killed Jackson. The propofol dose is irrelevant. The only thing that matters is observing and monitoring one's patient. Murray, by apparently failing to perform these two items, was truly reckless and inexcusable.

In conclusion, giving multiple drugs with the well-known potential to stop breathing, failing to remain in observation, and failing to use a pulse oximeter are all clear predictors of a bad outcome. Although he may not have intended to kill Jackson, Murray clearly caused Jackson's death involuntarily. The only thing more reckless Murray could have done was taking Jackson up in an airplane and pushing him out without a parachute.

What would have prevented Jackson's death? A knowledgeable, conscientious physician who both watched and monitored his oxygen—at the very least—absolutely would have. A brain monitor would have measured the propofol effect, thereby preventing a dose that stopped Jackson's breathing.

PART 2

*Five Things You MUST Know
Before Anesthesia*

Chapter 6

Things You MUST Know
Before Anesthesia

The twenty-first century is clearly the Information Age. The Internet continues to be a powerful force for spreading the word. For instance, many of you may have already read about my pioneering anesthesia from www.drfriedberg.com or www.GoldilocksFoundation.org. Meanwhile, the printed word still has the power to move, to inform, to inspire, and to educate. In fact, I wrote this book to expose the problems with twentieth century anesthesia care along with the corresponding solutions and how to best obtain those solutions for your *twenty-first* century anesthesia experience.

You probably understand that change of any sort is the most difficult thing anyone can ever hope to accomplish. For those who might be unfamiliar with it, here is the Serenity Prayer.

My thoughts for today, as I think them every day before commencing my crusade to change the world:

Grant me the **serenity** to accept things that cannot be changed,

The **courage** to change the things that must be changed,

And the **wisdom** to tell one from another.

No one can be more concerned with your well-being than you. It is not enough to assume that the "doctor knows best." Your surgeon is charged with your preoperative evaluation, performing your surgical procedure, and evaluating your postoperative recovery from your surgery. After your preoperative evaluation, your anesthesiologist's principle duty is to get you through your surgery without allowing you to die—that's your short-term care.

As long as you have a heartbeat and blood pressure upon your arrival to the recovery room, it is unusual for your anesthesiologist to see you again. Exceptions to this rule are some surgery centers and most office-based surgery. How well you function after you go home from the surgery facility is the long-term consequence of your short-term care!

You have to live with the long-term consequences of your short-term care!

The Five Things You MUST Know Before Anesthesia

The goal of my Goldilocks Foundation is to raise your need to understand why you must get over going under and why your brain, your most precious asset, is at risk for any surgery requiring anesthesia. Specifically, there are five Things You MUST Know Before Anesthesia:

1. Measuring the Wrong Thing (20th Century Anesthesia) versus Measuring the RIGHT Thing (21st Century Anesthesia)
2. The Obstacles in Your Path
3. Why You Have Pain after Surgery
4. Ketamine, the Fantastic Drug That Keeps You from Feeling Pain
5. You *DO* Have the Power to Get Goldilocks Anesthesia for Your Surgery

Let's examine each of these five things in further detail in the following chapters.

Chapter 7

The First Thing You MUST Know before Anesthesia—

Measuring the Wrong Thing (20th Century Anesthesia) Versus Measuring the RIGHT Thing (21st Century Anesthesia)

D id you know how your anesthesia is given to you *without* a brain monitor? Your anesthesiologist will rely on your preoperative evaluation to formulate a best guesstimate of how much drug to give you to start your anesthetic. The starting point for this dose will be your age and body weight. Why? Those numbers are the easiest ones to get.

Other things *factored* into the decision will be your prescription drug history, drug allergies, history of smoking and alcohol use, illicit or "street" drug use, herbal supplements, history of hepatitis or asthma, previous anesthesia experience(s) (like prolonged wake-up time, postoperative nausea and vomiting (PONV), history of motion sickness, and your general physical condition.

Mary's story shows the difference between twentieth century anesthesia and Goldilocks twenty-first century anesthesia:

Mary was a forty-three-year-old who had liposuction with general anesthesia. Afterwards, she was groggy and sick to her stomach. She threw up for three days after surgery despite being given drugs to prevent this.

She returned for additional liposuction, but because of her previous experience, she wanted a different kind of anesthesia. She received the Friedberg Method of Goldilocks anesthesia—brain-monitored propofol ketamine intravenous sedation. She awakened clear-headed without hearing, feeling, or remembering any of her surgery. She was not at all sick to her stomach, despite not *getting any drugs to prevent postoperative nausea and vomiting (PONV).*

One of the biggest factors influencing your brain's response to my anesthetic drugs is your genetic makeup or how your liver will breakdown my drugs. Studies have told me there is as great as a nineteen-fold variation in the way your liver will perform this task for my favorite drug, propofol—the one now made infamous by Michael Jackson's avoidable death. Before you become unduly distressed about receiving propofol yourself, let me tell you that tens (if not hundreds) of millions of people have had propofol *safely* because someone was watching and monitoring them—two features apparently missing in Jackson's case.

Replacing thiopental (or Pentothal®), propofol became available in North America around 1989. Only as it became more widely used did the following qualities of this sleep drug become revealed. Propofol is a short-acting, powerful anti-nausea agent, an anti-oxidant, and (as the public recently learned from Michael Jackson) a "happy" drug.

I began using propofol for both putting you to sleep (induction) and keeping you asleep (maintenance) for surgery in March 1992. Most of my colleagues only used propofol for induction primarily because of its great cost. The vast majority of my Goldilocks anesthesia patients require between 25-50 units of propofol a minute to achieve brain sedation levels between BIS 60 and 75. The story of two patients' different experiences truly illustrates the importance of measuring what I am medicating—your brain!

Molly was an otherwise healthy sixty-two-year-old anesthesiologist who, preoperatively, told me the last time she had propofol she slept for two days—an almost unbelievable story! I gradually drifted her off to sleep and during the early part of the case needed to reduce her propofol to 2.5 units per minute to keep her brain response between BIS 60-75. That dose is <u>one tenth</u> of my lowest average dose, yet her brain was getting the desired effect.

After her six-hour surgery, I turned off the propofol, and she quickly awakened saying it was the best anesthetic experience she ever had. She didn't hear, feel, or remember a single thing, had no PONV or pain, and was quickly discharged to the aftercare facility without a problem.

Less than two months later, I had to anesthetize Lars,
an otherwise healthy fifty-eight-year-old originally from
Greenland. After gradually drifting him off to sleep, I
found I needed 150 units of propofol to keep him in the
same 60 to 75 percent range as Molly. This 150 unit per
minute propofol dose was <u>three times</u> my high average
for Goldilocks anesthesia patients and sixty times more
than Molly required for the same brain effect!

After his six-hour procedure, he awakened just as
promptly as Molly, also without hearing, feeling or
remembering a thing about his surgery and quickly
able to leave the office for his home again without PONV
or pain.

Most patients require 25-50 units a minute of propofol. Without a brain monitor, there is simply no way either of these two patients, one needing as little as 2.5 units and the other needing as much as 150 units, would have had such a smooth anesthetic experience as they did with a brain monitor.

Despite preoperative patient information gathering, the dose you get to start your anesthetic (i.e., the induction dose) remains your anesthesiologist's best guess. Getting you to sleep* quickly is in the best interest of the production pressure of the operating room schedule. (*Anesthesia is more than sleep. Sleep is the shorthand expression for loss of consciousness. Anesthesia includes non-responsiveness to painful stimulation in addition to loss of consciousness, but more about the "non-responsiveness" issue later.)

Putting you "out" quickly has two very important consequences:

1. **Often you stop breathing**, causing your anesthesiologist
   to "breathe for you."
2. **Your blood pressure also drops**, sometimes to danger-
   ously low levels, causing your anesthesiologist to give
   you a drug like ephedrine to raise your blood pressure
   back to safer levels.

Now you are no longer able to talk to your anesthesiologist
to let him/her know *how* asleep you are. How much anesthetic
drug should you continue to be given (i.e., your maintenance
dosing)?

From July 1975 through December 1997, I practiced my anesthesia with the commonly taught belief that changes in your heart
rate and blood pressure were a clue to how your brain responded
to the administered drugs. Because I knew this could not be the
entire information about your brain, I was obliged to give you
more anesthetic than I thought you needed for fear of not giving
you enough. This twentieth century belief system (i.e., the art of
the controlled overdose) is what Stanford University taught me
as well as what virtually every other anesthesia training program
through the country taught legions of my colleagues.

From my earliest anesthesia experiences to December 1997,
I witnessed the introduction of the EKG or electrocardiogram,
the automated blood pressure device, and the pulse oximeter.
No longer was your pulse the only way to diagnose dangerous,
treatable heart (cardiac) rhythms. The continuous display of your

EKG showed the problem if it was there! No longer did your anesthesiologist have to spend the time to check your blood pressure to decide if it was too low or too high. The automatic blood pressure device saves that all-important time. No longer did your anesthesiologist have to rely on the color of your blood to decide if your oxygen level was too low. The pulse oximeter audibly tells everyone in the OR when bad changes happen in your oxygen levels.

What happened for you? Knowing everything about your body from your neck *down* helped drop the anesthesia death rate from 1 in 10,000 to less than 1 in 250,000. Obviously, my anesthesia drugs medicate you from your neck *up*—your brain!

Once fewer people died from anesthesia, closer scrutiny began of the other results of anesthetic drugs. Problems still remained because some of you took a long time to wake up from anesthesia. Some of you woke up nauseated and vomiting (PONV). And some of you were in so much pain that strong narcotic type painkillers (i.e., morphine, Demerol,® or fentanyl) were necessary to treat it.

Another serious consequence of our controlled overdose routine was that some patients, especially those over fifty, woke up disoriented and delirious, while others experienced dementia. Delirium and dementia were long-term consequences of short-term care—heartbreaking to families and costly to them as well. But the hospital and anesthesiologist felt they did their "job" by not having you die from surgery!

Since practical brain monitoring did not exist in the twentieth century, other theories were advanced to explain these undesirable anesthesia outcomes. Also, the number of elderly having surgery in the late twentieth century was not nearly as large as it has become nowadays. Recently, a new anesthesia society has even emerged to deal with the problems of anesthesia in the elderly: the Society for the Advancement of Geriatric Anesthesia (SAGA).

Until the 1996 FDA approval of practical brain monitoring, one had to have the *serenity* to accept the less desirable outcomes of twentieth-century anesthesia practice. I want to give you the *courage* to create the force for the twenty-first-century change in anesthesia practice and the *wisdom* to know why it must happen!

You have to live with the long-term consequences of your short-term care!

Chapter 8

The Second Thing You MUST Know before Anesthesia—

The Obstacles in Your Path

Your anesthesiologist, his native language, training, beliefs, and experiences. There are almost as many reasons physicians choose to practice anesthesia as there are physicians practicing this medical specialty. One of the most common reasons is that anesthesia does not *appear* to demand the level of doctor-patient communication as primary care or surgery. Often, the apparent minimal need for communication skills is a reason some physicians who are not native English speakers enter anesthesia (exceptions to this rule are the leaders in the field who actually enjoy speaking either to patients or to professional postgraduate educational meetings).

After your primary care physician chooses to send you for evaluation for a possible surgery, your surgeon will be the next physician you will have to communicate with on your way to the operating room. Ultimately, you will need to communicate with your anesthesiologist who likely has chosen this specialty because of the (erroneous) perception of the minimal communication that needs to happen.

The next obstacle you will encounter is embodied in the tongue-in-cheek definition of an anesthesiologist: *the one who is half-awake who keeps the patient half-asleep while the patient is being half-murdered by the half-witted.* Parenthetically, surgeons tend to only recall the first part of this sardonic definition.

Your anesthesiologist is a very hardworking physician and is often very fatigued not only by the hours of work but also by the stress of watching over you, keeping you from harm during surgery, and ensuring you wake up afterwards.

Because anesthesia is a mental activity that takes place inside your head, it is the surgeon who receives the glory for the physical action of the surgery. Almost always at the end of a surgery, the surgeon hears the compliment, "Nice job" or "Good work." Compliments to the anesthesiologist are rare.

Most anesthesiologists would confirm my experience. Often the only time "anesthesia" is mentioned is because of a negative outcome—you took too long to wake-up, threw up, or had severe pain after surgery. Positive reinforcement or "getting stroked" is a very rare part of the anesthesiologist's day.

On the remuneration issue, Medicare (and many insurance companies) pays about 33 cents on the dollar for anesthesia services and between 60 to 80 cents on the dollar for surgical services. The reasons for this disparity are beyond the scope of this book. Suffice it to say, anesthesia services are undervalued compared with surgical ones.

So anesthesiologists don't talk well with patients; they're tired, overworked, and underpaid. *What's so great about giving anesthesia?* you might ask.

There is also a tremendous adrenalin surge from "cheating" death in major surgery. If you were critically sick and had to have surgery, I often pictured myself standing between you and the entrance to the pearly gates, thinking, *"Not on my shift."*

As a younger anesthesiologist, I relished the challenge of keeping a critically ill patient alive through a perilous surgery. As I matured in my practice, the thrill of being an "adrenalin junkie" wore thin. Caring for patients in the OR is a tremendous and rare responsibility. I can control when you go to sleep, when you wake up, when you will or will not breathe, how much fluid you will get, and how many drugs (and what kind) you will receive.

Anesthesiologists love control. However, patients appear to defeat our best efforts. For example, I cannot control the emotional baggage you bring with you to your surgery. Like me, you may have been traumatized by your previous experiences with anesthesia and surgery. You may have lost a close family member during surgery. You may have been socialized to believe that all surgery means suffering in pain afterwards.

The insight of my inability to control your emotional baggage was one of the great "Aha" moments in my career. Preoperatively, I offer you concrete information about why this anesthetic experience will be different from others in your past. As an empathetic anesthesiologist, I regularly offer to hold your hand while you drift off to sleep. Lucy's story illustrates this point especially well:

As a young surgery assistant, Lucy had watched me give my Goldilocks anesthesia for half a year before deciding to have it when she had her nose fixed by her surgeon. The case went well, and she awakened and went home without any problems like PONV, pain, or prolonged wake-up time.

Four years later, she decided again to have my Goldilocks anesthesia for her breast augmentation. However, something was very different. Despite having seen other patients of mine undergo breast augmentation and awaken without pain, she was terrified she was going to be in pain.

No amount of my reassurance was enough to help her get past this mental hurdle. Sure enough, after she awakened, she proceeded to experience PONV even though she was not in pain. Later she admitted to me that she just could not get the fear of pain out of her mind before surgery. She failed to get over going under.

Same patient, same anesthetic, yet a different outcome. Why? My drugs cannot control the emotional baggage brought to surgery. Presented with the same situation today, I would recommend relaxation CDs like the ones I used to help get calmer before my hip replacement surgery.

You cannot expect to get your brain monitor demand met when you are on a gurney waiting to go down the hall for your surgery. This conversation absolutely must happen before you are even admitted to your surgical facility—whether that is a hospital, a surgery center, or your surgeon's office.

When you are trying to convince your anesthesiologist that you want a brain monitor for your surgery, first give some understanding before asking to be understood. Showing some understanding and empathy for the life of your anesthesiologist is likely to be the most effective tool in disarming skepticism and resistance to change.

You might begin by saying, "I know the surgeon is supposed to be the hero, but I want you to be my *anesthesia hero*. How many hours have you been working? How are you sleeping? Do you feel like you need a vacation or feel charged up for giving my anesthesia?"

Almost immediately, you have transformed your anesthesiologist from an impersonal service provider into a feeling human being. You have given something better than money—positive feedback by showing some understanding about the issues in his/her life.

You have to live with the long-term consequences of your short-term care!

Chapter 9

The Third Thing You MUST Know before Anesthesia—

Why You Have Pain after Surgery

Anesthesia is more than sleep. Sleep is the shorthand expression for loss of consciousness. Anesthesia includes non-responsiveness to painful stimulation in addition to loss of consciousness.

Patient movement in response to surgery pain has long been the defining goal for your anesthesiologist. Have you ever heard the expression, *"Runs around like a chicken without a head?"* To understand the full meaning of this expression is to know your brain is not necessary to generate movement in your body.

Without a brain monitor, it is impossible for me to tell if any movement you might make during surgery is caused by a signal from your brain or one from the spinal cord in your neck. A brain signal might mean you are beginning to awaken and need more propofol. A neck signal has nothing to do with the wakefulness of your brain, but calls for more local anesthesia by your surgeon!

Without a brain monitor to make the call (brain vs neck movement), I would be forced to treat every movement you might make as if it was a sign of you starting to awaken. Can you see how this confusion would force me to always overmedicate as I am unable to tell the difference? Routine overmedication is the main reason some of you take a long time to wake up after anesthesia.

Around the mid-1940s a drug that revolutionized anesthesia was introduced—curare. This drug paralyzes you, making it impossible for you to move. Believe it or not, shortly after the introduction of curare there was great debate within the anesthesia community about whether or not curare also blocked nerve communication in the brain—like keeping you from feeling pain.

To settle the debate, one brave anesthesiologist volunteered to have his carpal tunnel surgery done under curare. When he "awakened," he described every detail of the operation and the conversation during his surgery. That account did not prevent generations of anesthesiologists from using curare (and newer, curare-like drugs) during surgery to prevent patient movement. The practice of trying to look good to the surgeon (and nursing staff) opened the door for "anesthesia awareness."

Because of the routine practice of the art of the controlled overdose, anesthesia awareness happens only about once or twice in a thousand patients (about 0.1 of 1 percent). Recent studies have shown an 82 percent decrease in this already rare problem when a twenty-first century guide—a brain monitor—is used. Conversely, reviewing the anesthesia records of patients who have had anesthesia awareness, many showed no changes in either heart rate or blood pressure (now discredited twentieth century guides to anesthesia dosing).

What century of anesthesia practice do you want for your surgery—twentieth or twenty-first? The answer is obvious; measuring is better than guessing! Without a brain monitor, you are guaranteed to be overmedicated!

But if overmedication prevented you from having pain after surgery, why then do so many patients require powerful, narcotic pain medicines? Anesthesiologists "understand" this as the *wind-up phenomenon.*

During surgery with traditional general anesthesia, pain signals continue to arrive in your brain, winding it up as it were, but the anesthetic stupefies or dopes up your brain so it cannot make a response. Once the general anesthetic wears off in recovery, your brain cries out seeming to ask, "Who was hurting me while I was asleep and helpless? Ouch!"

Powerful, narcotic-type painkillers like morphine, Demerol,® or fentanyl are often given to you in response to your need. The side effects of these drugs often include PONV for which still more drugs called anti-emetics or anti-nausea medications are prescribed. These drugs sometimes have their own side effects and, even worse, fail to stop you from vomiting. Fortunately, the "nifty fifty" is the answer to keeping you from feeling pain during your surgery.

Chapter 10

The Fourth Thing You MUST Know before Anesthesia—
Ketamine, the Fantastic Drug That Keeps You from Feeling Pain

I n the 1950s, postoperative pain was treated with powerful narcotic painkillers like morphine or meperidine (Demerol®). Too often, your pain was *under*treated for fear of producing narcotic addiction and the all-too-real problem of accidental *over*treatment. Too much narcotic will stop your breathing and kill you.

There was no Narcan® (narcotic reversal drug) or pulse oximetry until much later than the 1950s. The 1950 researchers thought if another class of drugs could be developed to stop your pain without depressing (or stopping) your breathing, your post-op pain would be better treated with *neither* under- nor overtreatment.

The first class of drugs those researchers explored was the phencyclidines. The parent compound, phencyclidine phosphate, was marketed as Serenyl® by ParkeDavis in 1958 but was quickly withdrawn from the market because of undesirable side effects (i.e., hallucinations). Later, as it became a street drug, phency-clidine phosphate became better known by the initials, PCP.

The researchers did not give up quickly on this class of compounds. About six years later they began experimenting with a modified PCP molecule, ketamine (marketed as Ketalar®), which received FDA approval for use in people in 1971. Ketamine, like its predecessor, was introduced as the silver bullet, the complete, total intravenous (IV) agent—meaning no other agents needed for anesthesia.

Unfortunately, some of the first patients to receive ketamine for their anesthesia were women having elective termination of pregnancy, as abortions were delicately referred to then. Picture the horrific PCP-like bad dreams (or hallucinations and dysphorias) these women experienced. Imagine how negatively the recovery room nurses felt about ketamine because of the wild, untreatable behavior of these women!

Ketamine quickly gained a reputation as a safe drug but one not very suitable for adult patients. (Quickly after its introduction, patients emphatically wanted to avoid receiving this drug. So bad was ketamine's reputation that anesthesiologists coined the code word "dissociation" to keep patients from learning they were about to receive ketamine.)

Ketamine did become popular in children's burn units, especially for the extremely painful dressing changes. In 1975, during my anesthesia specialty training, I was introduced to using small doses of ketamine prior to positioning elderly patients for spinal anesthesia for pinning their fractured hips.

It turns out that neither the very young nor the very old were particularly susceptible to ketamine-produced nightmares.

The veterinarians soon noticed ketamine. Sometimes the drug is called cat or horse tranquilizer. The vets quickly discovered it was nearly impossible to kill an animal, even if the body weight dose was more than twice the recommended amount. Also, the animals did not complain about bad dreams. In conclusion, ketamine is a very safe drug, but one that many anesthesiologists have avoided for use in surgery, even to this day!

Sometime during the mid-1970s, Dr. Charles Vinnik, a Las Vegas plastic surgeon, began tiring of listening to his patients cry out when he injected local anesthesia under Valium® and Demerol® sedation. Even though his patients had amnesia for the experience, their cries were distressing to the OR staff too. He asked his anesthesiologist if there was anything else he could use that would eliminate the distressing reactivity of the patients. Ketamine was suggested.

Through trial and error, Vinnik came upon a dose of ketamine, which was formulated independent of your body weight to prevent you from feeling pain after you were rendered sleepy from Valium.® Although Vinnik published his secret to using ketamine (i.e., sleep first, then dissociation) *without* the dreaded hallucinations or dysphorias, his 1981 paper appeared in the plastic surgery literature. Vinnik's secret lay largely unnoticed in the anesthesia community until I heard him speak in Newport Beach in December 1991 and subsequently visited his Las Vegas office operating room in March 1992.

I considered Vinnik's use of ketamine potentially useful for you but not the very long hangover from Valium.® I believed that propofol might be a better fit for this purpose but could find nothing in the anesthesia literature to support what I thought was a reasonable extension of Vinnik's concept of *"sleep first, then dissociation."* My first fifty cases were my best guess to improve your care. By the fall of 1992, I realized I had solved both problems many of you were having after surgery—throwing up and pain! Since then, I have been on a mission to help every surgery patient get better anesthesia care.

In the 1990s, ketamine became a drug of abuse, a rave drug and later lumped together with Rohypnol® ("roofies") & GHB (*gammahydroxybutyrate*) as date rape drugs. You may be beginning to sense the enormous public, to say nothing of the professional, resistance I met trying to promote the use of ketamine for surgery! Over the past two decades of my advocacy, that resistance has begun to wane as more of my colleagues tried the 'nifty fifty' and were successful using my approach for anesthesia.

However, the measurement of the propofol effect in your brain allows the reproducible use of ketamine, which keeps you from feeling pain during your surgery. After five years of performing propofol ketamine (PK) intravenous sedation (the Friedberg Method), I learned about a recently FDA-approved monitor to measure the propofol effect in your brain. My surgeons kept clamoring for a less expensive way to administer propofol. The brain monitor appeared to offer more promise than my previous efforts with midazolam (Versed®) premedication.

Using a brain monitor with propofol ketamine is what I call the Friedberg Method of Goldilocks anesthesia. In many third-world countries, ketamine infusions are still performed in the way the drug was originally marketed. Now that propofol has become very inexpensive, more anesthesia providers from third-world countries have accessed my websites to obtain information with which to execute my paradigm for Goldilocks anesthesia.

Ketamine, ironically, turned out to be the perfect adjuvant drug, not the complete and total intravenous agent its makers originally intended it to be, at least in the Western world. Goldilocks anesthesia is less expensive, safer, and simpler and gives better outcomes (i.e., no PONV and only Tylenol-type post-op pain).

With the ability to describe anesthesia outcomes by depth of anesthesia, the negative effects of anesthesia have been reported at BIS less than 45 on a 0-100 scale. Postoperative cognitive dysfunction (POCD) is the fancy doctor name for the Alzheimer's type of confusion seen more often in patients over fifty that I believe is a function of giving too much anesthesia. Delirium lasts hours, days, weeks, or months. Dementia is not transitory.

You have to live with the long-term consequences of your short-term care! Goldilocks anesthesia avoids the nefarious practice of routinely overmedicating you for fear of under-medicating you. Goldilocks anesthesia is always just the right amount, not too little or too much!

Here is my personal story with the "nifty fifty" of ketamine I received for my own hip replacement surgery:

———————————

It's obvious to all, if one wants to keep one's horses, close the barn door before they depart, not afterwards. It should be equally obvious for the issue of control of postoperative pain. It's far better to prevent pain from occurring than to treat it after it happens.

For the past eighteen years (and 5,000 patients), I have been giving 50 mg ketamine three minutes PRIOR to the stimulation of the injection of local anesthetic to the surgical field for elective cosmetic surgery, reporting minimal post-op pain with unprecedented PONV rates (0.6 percent) WITHOUT anti-emetics in a high-risk patient population. One of fewer than twenty anesthesiologists to publish their work in the prestigious New England Journal of Medicine, Dr. Christian Apfel defined high-risk patients as non-smoking females with high incidences of previous PONV and/or motion sickness, and being treated with postoperative narcotics.

Understandably, many have been skeptical that cosmetic surgery might have little relevance to the surgical cases involving substantial postoperative pain. Sometimes I've wondered that myself. After all, cosmetic surgery "only" involves moving skin and fat.

Why should anyone care about the 50 mg ketamine I received for my total hip replacement in addition to my spinal anesthetic with brain-monitored propofol sedation? Every anesthesiologist with whom I shared my story asked the same question: "What could the ketamine possibly add to that anesthetic?"

I purposely went to a Southern California hospital to have an internationally renowned surgeon perform my surgery; I was confident with the large volume of previous hip replacements (about 5,000) with which to compare my care. When I faced my unavoidable need for a hip replacement, I was given the opportunity to validate if it was indeed "nifty to give fifty" for very painful surgery.

I doubt many of you would dispute that chopping off a thigh bone or a femoral head and reaming out the hip joint constitutes a significant surgical stimulus with a fair bit of postoperative pain. Add to the surgery itself the fact that I am a devout coward—partly why I became an anesthesiologist. I truly do not like pain and would much prefer to not have pain than to endure it and "tough it out." In short, I am not the best surgical candidate.

I was so anxious about my anesthesia that I wrote a three-page letter to the anesthesia service detailing my concerns about my care. I spoke to the person who assigned the cases to be sure to get a younger anesthesiologist who routinely monitored propofol sedation with a brain monitor. When I met my anesthesiologist on the morning of surgery (May 6, 2008), I was able to convince him to run my propofol between BIS 60-75 and administer 50 mg ketamine three minutes before my surgeon injected my skin before making his incision.

My surgeon typically performs five hips every Tuesday and Thursday. That 50 mg ketamine dose three minutes PRIOR to stimulation was the only difference between my anesthetic experience and the thousands of hips before mine.

After my 2 mg midazolam (Versed®) premedication wore off in the recovery room, I was transferred to the regular hospital floor room. I spent another forty-eight hours on the floor before being discharged. During my stay, I required nothing for pain! Consequently, I required nothing for postoperative nausea and vomiting (PONV) secondary to the narcotics (opioids) that are frequently used for postoperative pain management.

The floor nurses did not know about (or in other words were "blinded") to my little experiment. Some people may be willing to attribute the pain-free post-op course to the pre-op and post-op local anesthetic wound infiltration and the 100 micrograms of morphine in the spinal anesthetic, but the floor nurses told me they still had to medicate most of the other hip replacement patients for pain.

The most interesting aspect of my stay was the sponta-neous and unrehearsed comments from every floor nurse that came to check on me: "Dr. Friedberg, are you sure you had your surgery?" "We've NEVER seen a hip look like you!" "You don't LOOK like you've had surgery." *My explanation was that because of the pre-stimulation ketamine, no one had hurt me on the OR table.*

Surely enough, I actually had more discomfort on week two than my first postoperative week as my brain caught up to what had happened to my body. Personally, I did not suffer having my hip replaced and professionally, my experience validated my clinical experience of eighteen years and 5,000 patients who received my Goldilocks anesthesia for their cosmetic surgery! The cosmetic surgeons' nurses said precisely the same thing about my Goldilocks patients as the St. John's nurses did about how I looked (i.e., not like I had surgery).

The moral? It IS nifty to give fifty! As long as your brain activity is at BIS less than 75, there is nothing to lose and everything to gain for postoperative management. Bonus—if you can convince the surgeon to inject some lidocaine before the incision and drop some bupivicaine (Marcaine®) in the incision prior to closing, it is all the better for the patient.

For all who want to benefit from my minimal postoperative pain experience, take this checklist with you when you have your first visit with your surgeon, your first stop on your way to surgery. Ultimately, you will also need to ask your anesthesiologist the very same questions. The list not only has questions you must ask but also the answers you must receive.

Questions you must ask BEFORE surgery

1. Did you know anesthesia overmedication is routine *without* a brain monitor?

   Yes

2. Did you know anesthesia overmedication can be avoided *with* a brain monitor?

   Yes

3. Will I have a brain monitor* during my surgery?

   Yes. If they answer no, go where it's routine.

4. Did you know propofol is an anti-oxidant?

   Yes

5. Will Lidocaine be injected before my incision?

   Yes

6. Will Marcaine be left in my incision at the end of surgery?

   Yes

7. How soon after surgery will I wake up?

   Within minutes

8. How frequently does PONV** occur in your practice?

   Rarely

9. What about post-op shaking?

   Rarely

Brain monitor + (PK) Propofol Ketamine = Friedberg Method of Goldilocks Anesthesia. Goldilocks Anesthesia = not too much, not too little, always just the right amount

**PONV = Postoperative Nausea & Vomiting

Chapter 11

The Fifth Thing You MUST Know before Anesthesia—

You DO Have the Power to Get Goldilocks Anesthesia for Your Surgery

B y this point in our conversation, I trust I have helped you to solve the following six problems:

1. Understand that, without a brain monitor, you will absolutely be *over*medicated.

2. The risks of anesthesia overmedication are the flip side of the same coin of under-medication, namely failure to measure your brain during anesthesia.

3. The risks of anesthesia under-medication include anesthesia awareness with PTSD—*82 percent* of which can be prevented by using a brain monitor.

4. The risks of anesthesia *over*medication, especially if you are over fifty, include delirium, dementia, and

death—*virtually all* of which can also be eliminated by using a brain monitor.

5. Failure of anesthesiologists (and nurse anesthetists) to use a brain monitor include:

    a. fear of change

    b. fear of losing one's profession to a machine (the Luddite scenario)

    c. lack of belief a brain monitor is necessary

    d. failure to understand heart rate and blood pressure changes are unreliable signs of brain response to anesthetics

    e. lack of incentives—no additional anesthesia fee for using a brain monitor, surgical facility has to absorb (or "eat") the twenty-dollar cost of the disposable sensor

    f. lack of messaging from national organized anesthesia societies

    g. no force for change

6. The very best way for you to succeed (i.e., create the needed force for change) in having your brain monitored under anesthesia is to kick the surgical facility in their wallet!

Having anesthesia without a brain monitor shows a flagrant disregard for the value of your brain. Yes, a good surgical result is very important, but it is even *more* important you wake up from anesthesia with the same number of mental "marbles" that you started with! *Remember: You have to live with the long-term consequences of your short-term care!*

The bottom line is that you hold the "trump card" for change by refusing anesthesia care *without* a brain monitor. It will also be useful to send the administrator of the facility that would not use a brain monitor a note informing them about the loss of revenue from your surgery because of this deficiency. Anesthesia departments absolutely hate to hear from their administrators about any loss of revenue.

Please feel free to email me at drfriedberg@drfriedberg.com with any of your experiences—good, bad, or indifferent—that you've had after using the information contained in my book.

PART 3

A Patient's Bill of Rights

Chapter 12

The Nine Traits of an Empowered Patient

So, you've seen how traditional anesthesia practices don't work to your brain's advantage and have even had a taste of the solution. As you will see even more fully, Goldilocks Anesthesia is the answer for getting your anesthetic needs right every time. But before you can fully take advantage of the solution awaiting you, first you need to understand the critical role you play in securing your own safe surgery.

I wish I didn't have to write this chapter. I wish more anesthesiologists "got it," and I didn't have to be a burr in the side of the medical profession simply to get educated and passionate professionals to change. But I can't do it alone; this chapter is an effort to not only get you more informed about your own power as a patient—yes, you DO have power—but also to prepare you for the tenacious resistance you might well face from modern medical professionals.

Let's face it. Before you read my book, you might not have even known something like a brain monitor existed! Now I'm asking you to do something very challenging: asking your surgeon to support or encourage your anesthesiologist to use one!

It's challenging because many patients simply are intimidated by "making waves." So they tend to "go with the flow." We have been taught that "doctors know best," and it can be very difficult to question that logic when faced with an educated man or woman in a white lab coat. Add a wall full of framed doctoral degrees and a library of thick medical textbooks, and the intimidation factor goes up another few notches.

But if we are ever going to ensure that you and others in your circle of family and friends are to get over going under, you will need to be empowered to become a better patient. What do I mean by that? A better patient:

- *Has more confidence*
- *Knows what he or she is talking about*
- *Isn't intimidated by a stethoscope and lab coat*
- *Argues rationally, not emotionally*
- *Is more concerned with his or her health than the doctor's feelings*

Can you see how being a better patient challenges your medical professional to be a better doctor? Doctors are busy and face mounting pressures from a variety of fronts; it can be easy to slip into old habits and simply do things as they've always been done. But then someone like you comes along and challenges them to think differently and, guess what? *They will think differently.*

But only if you nudge them to. And that's our goal in this chapter. Here is where I introduce *the Nine Traits of an Empowered Patient*.

The First Trait of an Empowered Patient: *Passion*

Although it might sound odd (at first) to hear the word "passion" associated with medical care, you absolutely have to be passionate enough about your own care to demand something different—or better. My hope is that by the time you finish this book you will be passionate enough about having your brain monitored during surgery that you will accept nothing less!

The Second Trait of an Empowered Patient: *Persistence*

You have to be persistent to obtain the medical care you're entitled to. When I say persistent, I mean that if one doctor isn't willing to give you what you want—based on careful logic and research—then you must be persistent enough to find a doctor who will. It sounds like I'm simply suggesting that you get a second opinion, but it may take a third and even a fourth opinion. Can you be persistent enough to do that?

The Third Trait of an Empowered Patient: *Courage*

Doctors can be intimidating, particularly to those who have never had surgery before and/or have never had a specific type of surgery. In the old days, you knew your doctor and trusted him or her to take care of you. With the way healthcare exists today, we often have only a few consultations with our surgeon before going under the knife; use this time wisely and don't be afraid to speak your mind!

The Fourth Trait of an Empowered Patient: *Confidence*

Knowledge is power (see below). The more knowledge you have, the better informed you are about not only your medical condition but the opportunities for treatment that exist. Maybe you'll never know more than your physician, but no one knows you better than yourself.

When you speak to physicians, speak with confidence. If you're wrong, they'll tell you. If you're really wrong, ask them to explain why. If it makes sense, do some research on your own to understand why.

The Fifth Trait of an Empowered Patient: *Information*

Know what you're talking about before opening your mouth. This book tells you everything you need to know about brain monitoring and the Friedberg Method of Goldilocks Anesthesia; bring it with you to your next consultation. Highlight pages, bookmark them, photocopy them—better yet, memorize them!

If you become emotional when confronting professional people, rehearse at home using the information you've discovered. The point is to come to any consultation with any medical professional prepared with enough information to make your point. That's the best you can do. If he or she still refuses to use a brain monitor, then see Trait #2: Persistence and go elsewhere.

The Sixth Trait of an Empowered Patient: *Understanding*

Doctors are not bad people—far from it. They are, like the rest of us, creatures of habit. Many of them have done things the same way for the entirety of their careers, so be understanding if there is a little blowback from your revolutionary (to them, anyway) suggestions!

The Seventh Trait of an Empowered Patient: *Open-mindedness*

Like being understanding, having an open mind will help you see things from your physician's point of view. Likewise, you must be passionate and persistent (and confident) enough to explain—calmly, rationally, and with plenty of supporting information—why your point is equally valid.

The Eighth Trait of an Empowered Patient: *Willingness to Learn*

Let's say that when you ask about using a brain monitor during surgery, your physician gives you several reasons why it's not a good idea. Rather than getting up and storming out, don't throw the baby out with the bathwater. Instead, offer a compromise; schedule a second consultation and ask for time to study his viewpoints. Go home and compare his suggestions with what you've learned in this book and, when you return, have a side-by-side comparison to show him that you've considered his opinion but want him to do the same and consider yours.

The Ninth Trait of an Empowered Patient: *Patience*

It can take time to find the right physician for you. It can even take time to convince the right surgeon to use a brain monitor during your surgery; be patient. The beauty of these nine traits is that they work both independently and in concert with each other. The more of these traits you possess, the more likely you are to have surgery with a brain monitor. And remember, that's our ultimate goal for you.

Parting Words about Becoming an Empowered Patient

At the end of the day, your health really is in your hands. In this country, we count on something called self-reliance (or literally relying on yourself). You visit medical professionals for their experience and expertise, but as anyone who's ever undergone routine surgery in this country can tell you, there are a million ways a surgery can go wrong.

With so many working pieces—busy days, the time of year, nurses, doctors, assistants, anesthesiologists, your vital signs, and existing conditions—very rarely does any surgery in this country go off without a hitch. Your job is to ensure that your medical practitioners have every tool they need to do the job right. The more prepared you are, the more confident you are as a partner in your healthcare, the more you can help your doctor do what's best for you.

Remember, you and your loved ones are who have to live with the long-term consequences of your short-term care.

Chapter 13

Eight Simple Tips on How to Talk to Your Doctor

You may think you don't need to read this chapter. You may reason that you already know how to talk to your doctor, and I'm quite certain that you do. But before you skip to the next chapter, just think for a minute about what you and your doctor have talked about in the past. Typically, it's your doctor doing all the talking and you doing all the listening, or at least nodding your head!

This chapter is an animal of an entirely different color. What I'm asking you to do in chapter thirteen is not just talk to your physician but actively confront him or her (if necessary). Are you prepared to do that?

Really? Most of us aren't even comfortable confronting our bosses, family members, neighbors, or spouses; things can get even trickier when we're trying to tell a smart, educated, six-figure professional that we know what's right for us. Is that something you feel comfortable doing with no additional training?

Ah, that's what I thought. So, what *does* it take to not just talk to your physician but, if necessary, confront him or her? I'm glad you asked! And what's more, I'm glad you asked *me*, in particular. Why? It's simple; I have spent my entire career confronting my colleagues and fellow physicians on a variety of matters when it comes to my specialty, anesthesia. So if there's one person who's comfortable confronting doctors, it's one of their own!

Seriously though, speaking frankly, honestly, and openly to your physician doesn't have to be as intimidating as it sounds. And it won't be, if you follow the *Eight Simple Tips on How to Talk to Your Doctor:*

The First Tip: *Don't Come Angry or "Loaded for Bear"*

The worst way to begin a confrontation—any confrontation—is with anger, frustration, and pent-up emotions. You and I both understand your concerns and why you may potentially be frustrated with what you perceive as stubbornness on your doctor's part, but he or she won't IF you begin the conversation on the wrong foot.

Here is a little trick: Start as if your doctor is going to agree with you. That's the outcome you want, right? So act as if you're going to get it and you will find yourself responding much more pleasantly from the outset of the conversation.

Now, this isn't necessarily to say that your doctor will agree to provide a brain monitor during surgery, but it won't be for your lack of trying or, for that matter, your lack of civility. There is nothing wrong with acting civil, even when—particularly when—things aren't going your way. When you are calm and rational—versus angry and emotional—you tend to think better, make better arguments, and come off as more reasonable; all of which help you plead your case with that much more authority.

The Second Tip: *Listen First, Talk Second*

One way to have a more effective conversation is to actively listen to what is being said. By active listening, I mean don't just remain quiet while your doctor is talking but actively listen to what he or she is saying *while* they are talking. There might be a very good, or at least a very particular, reason why your doctor refuses to make this particular concession on your behalf. Maybe he is old school, maybe she doesn't have enough research at hand to make a proper decision, maybe he is bowing to political (or even peer) pressure; you'll never know the real reason for his or her refusal if you don't listen to your doctor's explanation.

Again, this isn't to say that listening alone will solve the problem. A "no" is still a "no" no matter how carefully you listen for it or hear it said. However, the best kinds of conversations are those where both parties understand each other; better listening always leads to better understanding.

The Third Tip: *Stay Calm*

No matter what, stay calm! No matter what you feel like doing, stay calm! No matter what you feel like saying, stay calm! No matter what your doctor says, stay calm! No matter what your doctor does, stay calm! Seriously, stay calm! I know it's not always easy, but it's always a valuable negotiating tool. Calm people:

- *Make better decisions*
- *Say smarter things*
- *Are able to override their emotions and tap into their rationality*
- *Make better arguments*
- *Take disappointment in stride*

Remember, the only thing your doctor can say is *"No, dear patient, I won't use or support the use of a brain monitor while administering anesthesia during your operation."*

He can't say, *"I hate you!"* He can't say, *"You're a horrible person!"* She can't say, *"I won't because you're stupid!"* All he or she can say is *"No,"* and as long as you have a backup plan for that (See Tip #8), there's no reason to get upset about your doctor's response.

The Fourth Tip: *Stay Calmer*

If you think you're staying calm, stay calmer. I'm serious about this. Being calm is so essential I'm using it for not one but two tips because, well, it's just that important!

The Fifth Tip: *Make Points, Don't Score Them*

This isn't a competition; it's not about who scores the most points but who makes them. In other words, don't try to trump your doctor with lots of medical mumbo jumbo if it's not in pursuit of a valid, meaningful point. That's why I recommend that you bring this book along. Highlight the most salient points, the research on over-anesthesia and its dangers, and the simplicity, cost, and effectiveness of brain monitors and (if necessary) quote them verbatim to your doctors. Those are the points you should be making, not worrying about who's shouting the loudest!

The Sixth Tip: *Agree to Agree—Or Disagree*

Going into any conversation with your doctor, know that there are two (and only two) resolutions: either you get what you want or you don't. It's that simple. What do you want? A simple twenty-dollar sensor connected to a brain-monitoring device during routine surgery. What will you accept? Nothing less than what you want!

Trust me, I'm the last guy to advocate patients making unreasonable demands on busy, overworked doctors; they have it hard enough. But I'm all for you making a simple, reasonable, and rational demand that you have every right to make—and that is within every doctor's power to approve. So, there's no reason to become emotional or upset; you either get what you want or you don't. If your physician agrees to include a brain monitor during anesthesia, great; you agree. If he doesn't agree, then you disagree—and look elsewhere for a more understanding physician.

The Seventh Tip: *Don't Burn Your Bridges*

Remember, our very first tip is to never go into a confrontation loaded for bear. It's always best to remain calm, open, rational, and as unemotional as possible. I know this can be challenging when we're talking about your health, but remember that rather than become an adversary your doctor can become a powerful ally in your healthcare.

Even if he doesn't agree to offer you the use of a brain monitor during surgery, he may recommend someone—someone very good—who will. The point is, you WILL never know if you burn a bridge, call your doctor lots of names and storm out of the room without discussing your available options first.

The Eighth Tip: *Have a Walk-Away Point*

Everyone needs a walk-away point when negotiating. That point where they've reached a deal breaker and can't take it anymore. For you, it should be fairly simple: either you get what you want or you don't. However, it's important to be clear about what you want and reasonable about how to get it.

For instance, maybe your doctor doesn't understand the brain monitor and wants to learn more about it. Don't take this as a definite no, but instead commit to hearing his opinion after he learns more. If after doing more research, your physician still refuses to offer you a brain monitor during surgery; that is your walk-away point. Walking away too soon can be as damaging as not walking away at all, so pick your walk-away points carefully.

Parting Words about the Eight Simple Tips on How to Talk to Your Doctor

As you can see, none of these talking points is difficult or unreasonable on its own. The main variable in all these tips is how you go about the process of communicating with your physician. These eight tips work best when you practice some common sense while using them.

As always, be patient, be calm, be reasonable, be rational, and (above all else) be respectful. You won't get anywhere by trying to bully, coerce, or shout down your physician!

Chapter 14

Doing the Research—
Five Steps for Coming Prepared

When people talk to me about their doctor, or even physicians in general, they tend to get rather emotional, which is only natural. Think about it; going to the doctor isn't something we do every day, and when we do, it's normally NOT because we're feeling healthy! So in addition to NOT feeling very good, you're faced with the prospect of a surgical procedure that will involve nurses, a surgeon, an anesthesiologist, various support staff, and perhaps an overnight or even extended hospital stay, to say nothing of the procedure itself; none of which is very appealing.

People usually experience a strong emotional response to surgery, in particular. In fact, for many, the thought of going under the knife—or simply going under anesthesia—is a VERY emotional experience. Unfortunately, while emotion is healthy for the soul, it's often not a great bargaining chip! When we try to reason based on emotion, we often fail and instead resort to begging, borrowing, or even berating our doctors to get what we want. However, none of those options seems likely to win you the desired result you are ultimately looking for.

This chapter is designed to help take the emotion out of the equation when you suggest to your doctor that he or she use a brain monitor during anesthesia while undergoing your next surgical procedure. Reason trumps emotion in nearly every intelligent discussion, and the conversation you have with your doctor over this topic is important enough to leave your emotion at home and pack plenty of reason, logic, and good, old fashion facts instead! To help you, here are *Five Steps for Coming Prepared* to your next doctor's visit.

Step 1: *Make Up Your Mind*

What, exactly, do you want to achieve? Be specific, and go to your doctor with a laundry list of items you want. After reading it, sum it all up by adding, *"Oh, yeah, and I'd also like a brain monitor during anesthesia!"*

Remember why you're here and what you want to accomplish; focus on one goal at a time. If you have multiple goals, have multiple office visits or make sure your doctor has enough time to cover them all. I always recommend making a specific office visit simply to bring up and confirm that you will be having a brain monitor during surgery; this is the solution you want and the one that the discussion should center around.

Step 2: *Do Your Homework*

If you have a doctor's appointment next Thursday afternoon at three, you must start building your case for a brain monitor during anesthesia now, NOT next Thursday at 2 P.M.! Spend some time each day building your case. Again, use this book as a reference, but don't stop there. The Internet, the library, even the hospital's resource center are all valuable places where you can backup my information with up-to-the-minute resources as well.

I try to keep my website, www.drbarryfriedberg.com, updated, so start there. You can print out pages, copy statistics, or merely quote me! The important thing is to bring some information with you to backup your argument if—and quite possibly when—your surgeon or anesthesiologist balks at the idea of using a brain monitor.

Step 3: *Prioritize Your Argument*

Doctors want to know what matters; you want to know what matters too. That's why it helps to prioritize your argument when getting ready to talk to your surgeon. After all, the more you can convince him or her that this brain monitor is important to you, the more likely he or she will use it during your upcoming surgery. So, list the many reasons why you want a brain monitor:

- *You have concerns about nausea after surgery.*
- *You're worried about the risks of over- or under-anesthesia.*
- *You're concerned about potential memory loss as a result of over-anesthesia.*

- *You want your brain signals to be monitored under anesthesia, not just your heart rate and blood pressure.*

Now, look at your list and prioritize it. In other words, why are you MOST interested in having your brain monitored during surgery? Look at the list again and rearrange it in order of your biggest concern to your smallest concern. After careful consideration, your revised list might look like this:

- *You're concerned about potential memory loss as a result of over-anesthesia.*
- *You have concerns about nausea after surgery.*
- *You want your brain signals to be monitored under anesthesia, not just your heart and blood pressure.*
- *You're worried about the risks of over- or under-anesthesia.*

Regardless of what your list looks like, this step is important because writing something down helps commit it to memory. You can even bring it in with you and use it as a tool as you discuss your various concerns with your surgeon.

Step 4: *Make Your Case*

It can help make the process more realistic if you actually write down the case you're trying to state. In addition to any printed pages you may want to bring with you or highlighted facts or figures (or even this book), take a blank sheet of paper and literally state your case.

You may say something like, "It's very important to me that I not be given too little sedation or too much. To make sure I get just the right amount, I'd like to use a brain monitor during this surgical procedure. Here are the reasons why…"

Or you may simply elaborate on Step 3 (see above) and flesh out some bullet points that rank by priority why you want a brain monitor used during surgery. The point isn't to write the great American novel, but instead to underscore for yourself what exactly it is you want and why, exactly, you want it; sometimes writing things like that down can help you focus on them more fully when it comes time to repeat them.

Step 5: *Practice Makes Perfect*

Although it may sound a little extreme to role-play your next doctor's office visit, if you are someone who doesn't handle confrontation well or gets really intimidated by your doctor, why not? Ask a friend, family member, neighbor, roommate, or coworker to be a "stand in" for your doctor and practice how the discussion might go. Don't just have your stand in say yes immediately either! Instead, encourage him or her to play devil's advocate and press you on why, exactly, you think a brain monitor is necessary.

This will force you to draw on your research and the four previous steps to fine tune the argument you hope to make when it comes time to actually have this discussion with a real, live physician.

Parting Words about Doing Your Research

Doctors are mainly scientists at heart. We deal in facts, figures, equations, and measurements and respond best when presented with a factual thesis versus an emotional plea. So come prepared with facts, be prepared to back them up and you may just be surprised by how willing your doctor is to hear your plea. And of course, if he isn't, go find someone who is!

Chapter 15
A Patient's Bill of Rights

W hat is the *Patient's Bill of Rights?*
Here you will find a summary of the Consumer Bill of Rights and Responsibilities that was adopted by the US Advisory Commission on Consumer Protection and Quality in the Health Care Industry in 1998. It is also known as the Patient's Bill of Rights.

The Patient's Bill of Rights was created to try to reach three major goals:

1. **To help patients feel more confident in the US health care system, the Bill of Rights:**
   - *Assures that the health care system is fair and it works to meet patients' needs*
   - *Gives patients a way to address any problems they may have*
   - *Encourages patients to take an active role in staying or getting healthy*

2. **To stress the importance of a strong relationship between patients and their health care providers**

3. **To stress the key role patients play in staying healthy by laying out rights and responsibilities for all patients and health care providers**

This Bill of Rights also applies to the insurance plans offered to federal employees. Many other health insurance plans and facilities have also adopted these values. Even Medicare and Medicaid stand by many of them. The eight key areas of the Patient's Bill of Rights are listed below.

1. Information for patients

You have the right to accurate and easily understood information about your health plan, health care professionals, and health care facilities. If you speak another language, have a physical or mental disability, or just don't understand something, help should be provided so you can make informed health care decisions.

2. Choice of providers and plans

You have the right to choose health care providers who can give you high-quality health care when you need it.

3. Access to emergency services

If you have severe pain, an injury, or sudden illness that makes you believe that your health is in danger, you have the right to be screened and stabilized using emergency services.

You should be able to use these services whenever and wherever you need them without needing to wait for authorization and without any financial penalty.

4. Taking part in treatment decisions

You have the right to know your treatment options and take part in decisions about your care. Parents, guardians, family members, or others that you choose can speak for you if you cannot make your own decisions.

5. Respect and non-discrimination

You have a right to considerate, respectful care from your doctors, health plan representatives, and other health care providers that does not discriminate against you.

6. Confidentiality (privacy) of health information

You have the right to talk privately with health care providers and to have your health care information protected. You also have the right to read and copy your own medical record. You have the right to ask that your doctor change your record if it is not correct, relevant, or complete.

7. Complaints and appeals

You have the right to a fair, fast, and objective review of any complaint you have against your health plan, doctors, hospitals, or other health care personnel. This includes complaints about waiting times, operating hours, the actions of health care personnel, and the adequacy of health care facilities.

8. Consumer responsibilities

In a health care system that protects consumers or patients' rights, patients should expect to take on some responsibilities to get well and/or stay well (for instance, exercising and not using tobacco). Patients are expected to do things like treat health care workers and other patients with respect, try to pay their medical bills, and follow the rules and benefits of their health plan coverage. Having patients involved in their own care increases the chance of the best possible outcomes and helps support a high quality, cost-conscious, health care system.

Chapter 16
The Nine Things You Should Ask Checklist

Once you recover from the shock that you have to undergo surgery, the nine essential questions you must ask your surgeon are a good starting point to get the Friedberg Method of Goldilocks anesthesia.

1. **Did you know anesthesia overmedication is routine *without* a brain monitor?**

   This is a leading question. Few surgeons have any concept of anesthesia beyond "my patients don't move when I work and they return to the recovery room alive." This question leads your surgeon to understand why you will be asking the next two questions. The answer to question 1 is YES.

2. **Did you know anesthesia overmedication can be avoided *with* a brain monitor?**

   This question lets your surgeon know you are not only aware of a potential problem but what can be done to avoid it. The answer to question 2 is also YES.

3. **Will I have a brain monitor during my surgery?**

   This question lets your surgeon know you want to avoid the risks of anesthesia overmedication—delirium, dementia, and even death. The answer to question 3 goes beyond YES. *If the answer is no, politely tell your surgeon your brain is too precious to you, and therefore you must go where it is a routine. Don't forget the facility administrator's letter, as well. Sample available for download @ www.drbarryfriedberg.com.*

4. **Did you know propofol is an anti-oxidant?**

   This question lets your surgeon know that you understand the difference between propofol and the stinky gases. The answer to question 4 is YES too.

5. **Will Lidocaine be injected before my incision?**

   This question lets your surgeon know you would prefer the nerves in your skin don't cause the wind-up effect in your brain during your surgery. The answer to question 5 is YES.

6. **Will bupivicaine (Marcaine®) be left in my incision at the end of the surgery?**

   This question allows you to discuss your desire to avoid narcotic painkillers if at all possible. The side effects of these drugs are PONV and constipation (neither of which are desirable after your surgery). The answer to question 6 is YES.

7. **How soon after surgery will I wake up?**

   This question ties back to avoiding anesthesia overmedication risks (delirium, dementia, and death) that you raised in questions 1, 2, and 3. The answer should be within minutes of surgery being finished.

8. **How frequently does PONV occur in your practice?**

    This question lets your surgeon know that you would like to avoid both types of drugs that cause this problem—the stinky gases and the IV narcotics. The answer to question 8 should be very rarely.

9. **What about post-op shaking?**

    This is a little insiders' knowledge. Goldilocks anesthesia patients rarely shake postoperatively. The answer to the last question is also very rarely.

Conclusion

By now you should be feeling very empowered about speaking with your physician and, best of all, getting what you want out of the conversation. Hopefully, you understand the difference between emotion and accusation and logic and reasoning—and which works best in a conversation this serious.

Why did I write this book? The reasons are many, and I have discussed them all already, but for the most part, it is my intention that you use this book as more than just a guide, but a tool; bookmark it, dog-ear it, highlight it, memorize it, and bring it with you on your next surgical consultation visit.

For too long, patients have felt like second-class citizens in the eyes of the medical profession. Many, in fact, have even foregone their own needs by placing a blind sense of trust in their physicians. I am not here to downgrade modern doctors or, for that matter, the medical profession itself. Most doctors are experts in their fields and as such deserve our respect.

But respect is earned, not given, and surgery requires a mutual commitment by both parties: surgeon and patient. When you're railroaded into decisions despite your protestations, when your best evidence and rational explanations for the safety and simplicity of a brain monitor are ignored, respect is hard to come by. But there's always a door to walk out of, and another surgeon to speak with. I hope by now this book has shown you not only to be respectful, but to demand respect as well.

In the end, the Friedberg Method of Goldilocks Anesthesia is about feeling just right—before, during, and after surgery. We have spent a fair amount of time together understanding why the proper amount of anesthesia is so critical and why monitoring the brain during surgery is just so important. Remember, it's up to you to get both the surgery and the anesthesia you deserve. You can look at this book as a field guide for how to do both, with respect both given and earned. Everything you need for better medical care in general, and a much better anesthesia experience in particular, can be found in this book.

Now all you have to do is use it!

A Message from Dr. Friedberg

W ho am I and why do I care so much about how much anesthesia you or one of your loved ones receives during your next surgery?

My name is Dr. Barry L. Friedberg, and my career is the medical practice of anesthesia. My formal anesthesia training was at Stanford (1975-1977) after which I passed my boards to become a Diplomate of the American Board of Anesthesiology or a board-certified anesthesiologist (1980).

To improve patient care, I pioneered the use of the automated blood pressure device (1979), Swan Ganz/cardiac output monitoring for critically ill patients (1981), and the pulse oximeter (1984) at my local Newport Beach, California hospital. I did these things in the face of fierce local resistance and without any personal financial gain. In fact, introducing modern technology at my facility actually cost me money.

After five years in open-heart surgery anesthesia, I moved to outpatient, or ambulatory, surgery-center anesthesia. I left the institutional setting of Newport Beach in 1991 and developed propofol ketamine (PK) anesthesia (the Friedberg Method) in 1992. PK was derived from Vinnik's Valium® ketamine anesthesia published in 1981 and further popularized by other plastic surgeons like Baker, Stuzin, and Ersek.

PK anesthesia (the Friedberg Method) was designed to maximize patient safety while imitating general anesthesia. Under PK anesthesia, patients do not hear, feel, or remember their surgical experience. Since 1993, I have practiced exclusively in the subspecialty of office-based anesthesia (OBA) for elective cosmetic surgery. Because of the unique challenges in the office-based setting, I saw a need for the education of my hospital-based colleagues who might choose a path similar to my own.

I founded the Society for Office Anesthesiologists (SOFA) in 1996 and merged it in 1998 with the Society for Office Based Anesthesia (SOBA), another non-profit, international educational society dedicated to improving patient safety. In 1997, I became the first anesthesiologist in Orange County, CA, to begin routinely monitoring my patients with a brain-activity monitor, significantly refining PK anesthesia as the Friedberg Method of Goldilocks Anesthesia. Many anesthesiologists expressed similar skepticism about brain activity monitoring that they had earlier expressed about the automated blood pressure device. As with earlier technological patient care advances I pioneered, I had no financial involvement with the brain monitor maker.

When Olivia Goldsmith, author of *The First Wives' Club* died in 2004, the need for a comprehensive textbook in the field of cosmetic surgery anesthesia became apparent. My reputation and extensive publications in the field made me the *first* choice among 40,000 US anesthesiologists to write this groundbreaking textbook.

Also, in 2004, I received a US Congressional award for contributing to the anesthesia safety of the Coalition's wounded soldiers in both Iraq and Afghanistan. The portability of PK anesthesia (the Friedberg Method) does not require the routine use of anesthesia machines and the large quantities of oxygen needed to run them. This small, highly mobile footprint reduced the military's logistical problems associated with transport and maintenance of anesthesia machines in the forward surgical units.

Cambridge University Press published my book, *Anesthesia in Cosmetic Surgery*, in April 2007 in English, followed by the book's Portuguese translation for Brazil in June 2009. Brazil performs the most cosmetic surgeries of any country in the world. Subsequent citations of my PK anesthesia articles are noteworthy because half of all the published journal articles are never referred to in later journal articles by other authors. However, my articles have been cited in over sixty *subsequent* journal articles. My articles have also been cited in twenty anesthesia textbooks including the prestigious 2010 *Miller's Anesthesia*.

In addition to the legal profession, the California Medical Board also recognizes me as a medical expert in anesthesia. My expertise has been lent to a number of peer-reviewed medical journals for review. I am also a contributor in several anesthesia and surgery journals.

From 1998 through 2008, I volunteered as Assistant Professor of Anesthesia at USC in Los Angeles and again from 2009-2010 as Associate Professor of Anesthesia at the University of California, Irvine.

I have also lectured to anesthesiologists and surgeons in the United States, Canada, Mexico, the Dominican Republic, Israel, Venezuela, Kuala Lumpur, Singapore and Dubai. Although these lectures for safer, simpler, cost-effective anesthesia with better patient outcomes are more often requested by surgeons rather than anesthesiologists.

I was also honored to give Anesthesia Grand Rounds in 2005 at the University of Southern California (USC), and, in 2009, at Los Angeles' prestigious Cedars Sinai Hospital. Most recently, the Biennial Pan Pacific Plastic Surgeon's meeting in Honolulu (January 2010) even removed a surgeon's lecture to make room on the schedule for mine.

None of this information really matters unless you understand that everything I do as an anesthesia professional, I do for you, the patient.

www.drbarryfriedberg.com